Children A
Mauric

Copyright Joseph
Clachan Publishing
26 Rathlin Road, Ballycastle,
Glens of Antrim, BT54 6AQ

Email: clachanpublishing@outlook.com
Website: http://clachanpublishing-com.
ISBN: 978-1-909906-59-4

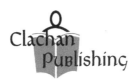

Children Are my Heroes

Maurice Savage

This book is dedicated to my late parents Jim and Mabel Savage
who unstintingly supported me in my ambition to study medicine and become
a doctor, to Anne, my wife, for her love and encouragement
despite the many absent hours when I disappeared
to write, and to my children
Mark,
Emily,
and Joanna
and their children,
as they follow their own dreams.

His Name is Today

We are guilty of many errors and many faults,
But our worst crime is abandoning the children,
Neglecting the fountain of life.
Many of the things we need can wait.
The child cannot wait.
Right now is the time his bones are being formed.
His blood is being made,
And his senses are being developed.
To him we cannot answer, "Tomorrow".
His name is Today.

Gabriella Mistral
Nobel Prize Winning Poet from Chile

Contents

Children are my heroes, (and parents deserve a medal.)

18. Difficult questions

Bigger questions, Is the surgeon any good? , When can I get out of here? , Does epo work on dogs? , Laughter, the best medicine, Aaron's hug, Relief and release, *Fit for anything*

The drummer, Sisters, Going home, A wedding present, The mitt of St Jude, Good memories

Prologue

Dreaming

Some nights I dream of the sick children I have looked after over many years. None are clearly recognisable, but I am in no doubt that they are patients once in my care. The surroundings are not in focus in these dreams. Sometimes there are glimpses of happy little faces, even cheeky, mischievous faces, rather than sad or frightened ones. Often, I see the pale, anxious, fearful faces of parents, their eyes searching mine for reassurance. I experience again the tension and adrenalin release as critical events unfold and stress crescendos. Next, it seems that I am involved in some intricate clinical procedure which, despite my total concentration, I cannot complete. I am trapped in a frustrating repetitive loop of ineffective activity. The dream is irrational and eventually fragments like breaking glass. I awaken feeling tense and frustrated, my heart pounding. It takes several moments to realise the dream is not real. I am not, after all, in the Paediatric Intensive Care Unit. There are no reassuringly regular bleeps from nearby cardiac or respiratory monitors, no soft wheeze from artificial ventilators, no antiseptic smell, no digital monitor screens, only the bedside clock radio with its fluorescent numbers confirming it is 3 or 4:30 a.m. There are no bright artificial lights, the room is in darkness. I am lying in the comfort of my own bed with my wife, Anne, sleeping soundly beside me.

I am filled with a great sense of relief. I don't, after all, need to initiate emergency resuscitation procedures or even to concentrate again on the meticulous technique of inserting a fine needle with its cannula into a tiny vein. I have no critical decisions to make. I dont, this time, need to calm my racing heart, collect my thoughts and mentally rehearse how best to clearly communicate distressing information to young parents. Parents who have been suddenly thrown into a crisis beyond any previous experience in their lives. A mother and father so terrified of what is happening to their most precious and loved son or daughter, that they will only remember a few of the sentences I speak, and perhaps only my first few words, if they are not positive.

Relieved, I turn over, adjust my pillow and lie thinking about families whose darkest days I have briefly shared. Days that stretched like eternity for them. I remind myself of the many children recovered to boisterous good health as I slowly drift off towards sleep.

On many occasions when people have suggested to me that being a children's doctor must be especially difficult and demanding, since my patients cannot describe their symptoms and are generally fearful of strangers and strange surroundings. I reply that adult patients may have similar characteristics and fears, but just do not act them out. I tend to deny any special diagnostic skill, knowing that winning a child's trust is the most important challenge.

Children may not be great at describing their symptoms but, conversely, they are not afraid to tell their doctor exactly what they think of them. There is usually no need to request feedback on performance, especially when it does not come up to a child's expected standard. A second attempt at a blood test is likely to be met with uninhibited protests. I know from personal experience that children have the unique ability to keep the most self-important doctor's feet on the ground and, long ago, I learned to expect and respect this capacity and refine my practical techniques in response. The great majority of sick children recover and bounce back to health. Most do not hold a grudge, are brave in adversity, easy to love and perceptive of kindness. They respond with some degree of tolerance, and even affection, for those nurses and doctors they come to know. To have received this trust is a very special reward.

Why, then, these recent dreams, when my hectic days of clinical practice are past? Perhaps it is a result of neglecting the traditional advice not to become too emotionally involved with patients.

Sometimes, after such a dream, I lie thinking about this, and conclude I could not have avoided such involvement with children and parents who demonstrated enormous courage and resilience. Perhaps the dreams come from a persisting, subconscious mourning for the children we could not save, despite the best efforts of the entire team. Buried memories surface on such occasions, of returning home with a heavy heart but fortunate to be rescued by the warmth of a loving family.

For now, I am asleep again.

2

1. Formative years

I was probably destined to become a paediatrician from the first day I walked onto a children's ward as a medical student. I was met by a tiny girl in a pretty dress, who reached a warm chubby hand to take mine. Without saying a word, she pulled me along the corridor towards the office.

"And what is your name?" I asked. In return, I received only a short shake of her head and a smile, which instantly stole my heart. Stopping, I knelt down, thinking she might not have heard what I had said, and gently asked again. It was then I saw that she was pointing at her throat. There was a plastic tracheostomy tube visible above the collar of her pink dress. It was held in place by two ribbons, attached on each side and tied together in a bow behind her neck. I realised she was unable to speak.

"Ah!" said the ward sister, peering out of her ever-open office door.

"I see our Becky has adopted you. She can spot an easy touch from a mile away."

Rebecca stuck out the tip of her tongue at her and skipped off. Sister shook her head benignly and smiled. I learned from her that Rebecca had been an in-patient for many months while surgeons tried to work out how to reconstruct a tight stricture in her windpipe: the trachea. The plastic "trachy" tube entered her windpipe below her larynx, the voice box, and below the obstruction in her airway, enabling her to breathe easily through it. She could make some sounds if she blocked the opening in the tube with her finger but, in reality, she had few problems communicating what she needed or wanted. Top of the list was company, friendship, attention, and affection from her favourite ward staff. This was readily given. I was lucky to briefly become included in those she favoured. I wished I had the ability to do something for her. That would take years of specialist training.

This first encounter with a child with what seemed to be an insoluble problem came towards the end of my years as a medical student, which had begun in the late 1960s with the study of Biomedical Sciences. Back then, one topic in particular dominated my interest.

Human Anatomy

The skeleton gazed out of its empty eye sockets at the 90 or so students, 25 of them female, all sitting uncomfortably on the ancient, tiered wooden benches. (Today the majority are likely to be women.) On that first day of a new semester he was dressed, for once, in a clean, starched white lab coat. A thin spiral of blue smoke drifted towards the roof of the lecture theatre from the long cigarette clamped between his grinning teeth. At precisely nine o'clock, the door to his right burst open. The impressive figure of the distinguished, white-haired professor swept in, white coat-tails flying in his wake. It was unlikely that the coat could have been buttoned across his ample front. Benignly, he took in the scene. He chose to ignore our flagrant infringement of the No Smoking rule, except for a wry smile. With good humour, he welcomed us to his course and the day's lecture. He scrawled the title with chalk on the large blackboard, 'The Abdominal Cavity'. Then, turning to the audience again, he leaned on the wooden lectern and his florid features became serious.

"Ladies and gentlemen, later this morning, we will all be going to the dissection room. We regard it a sacrosanct area and, by law, only medical students and specifically designated academic staff are permitted to enter. This will be one of the most important and memorable moments of your careers. You will see there, on each dissection table, a cadaver, a human body, covered by a white sheet. The most important thing you will learn today is not about the contents of the abdomen. It will be to learn to treat these bodies with respect. When these individuals were alive, they voluntarily decided to donate their bodies to medical science. They have given you a unique gift which you are honour-bound not to waste."

He paused for us to assimilate this injunction.

"You will be allocated in groups of six or eight to a table at which you will work, under supervision, for the next 18 months. It will be an experience which will transform you from ordinary university students into medical students and, ultimately, doctors.

At the end of that period, I expect you to have an intimate and detailed knowledge of the human body. No matter which branch of medicine you

4

aspire to practice, an understanding of the relevant body structure will be crucial."

So we were inducted into a tradition of medicine which stretched back to the days of Hippocrates, through history to Leonardo da Vinci's anatomical studies and to Versalius, the father of dissection.

The Professor then turned to his chosen topic for the day. For almost an hour, his passion for his subject and his unique style enthralled us. Disdainful of overhead slides, the forerunner of digital powerpoint images, he explained internal abdominal anatomy with layer upon layer of multicoloured chalk diagrams, drawn with an artistic flourish, directly onto the blackboard.

Later, in the dissection room, we watched warily as the white sheet was drawn back by our anatomy demonstrator, a trainee surgeon, to expose a male cadaver. After a few words of encouragement, he made the first long incision from the lower end of the breast bone down to the pubic symphysis. No one fainted, although some sat down on the stools provided. My reaction was not one of horror, as might be expected. I found, instead, that I was fascinated as the internal organs were revealed. Our donor's body was grey, stiff and cold to the touch of my gloved hands. The pungent smell of formaldehyde in the preservative was a distraction never to be forgotten. I was to find a particular satisfaction in locating and identifying each organ, and dissecting their internal structure and connections. One afternoon, we were surprised to find in the forearm of our cadaver, a metal plate which had been used to repair a fracture, reminding us he once had an active life.

It was a few weeks later that we isolated the renal blood vessels travelling from the aorta to supply the kidneys, their drainage ureters descending to the bladder, and I first held a human kidney in my hands. This organ, its function and malfunction, would later preoccupy my professional life. By now, I was certain I had chosen the right career. Much later I came to realise this dead person was my first patient and one who taught me more than most others I would encounter.

The First Post Mortem

Although studies of the biomedical sciences were important because of their relevance to medicine, their delivery seemed divorced from any contact with the reality of illness or disease. The compulsory attendance at a post-mortem, as part of the anatomy course, was as close as we came to an actual patient. So, on one dull winter morning, the six or seven members of my dissection group filed into the cold morgue building on the nearby hospital site. Apprehensive, we were welcomed by a grey-haired mortuary attendant and led into a cavernous room with a damp ceramic floor and tiled walls. He wore a white lab coat and protective trousers, tucked into white ankle-length rubber boots. Around his neck hung a loosely tied surgical mask. We were soon attired in the same uniform.

A bright cluster of overhead lights starkly illuminated a metal table on which we could discern the outline of the deceased person under a spotless green surgical drape. We stood silently along the wall, breathing in the pungent disinfectant-laden atmosphere, thinking of the stories previous students had related to us. A door to the side swung open, and the pathologist entered, followed by a police officer, who then stepped aside in deference.

"Good morning ladies and gentlemen," said the doctor, with a friendly smile.

"I am sure you have an idea of what I will be doing today, and will already have some experience of dissection of the human body. Nevertheless, you may find today's experience more daunting. If this is the case, and you feel you wish to leave, sit down for a minute, or get some fresh air, do not be embarrassed. You will not have been the first, or indeed the second or third student, to feel this way."

I assumed that this was a forensic post-mortem, and the policeman was present as a matter of procedure to confirm that any relevant findings were accurately recorded. The policeman in question looked barely older than us.

I muttered to the person standing, grim faced, beside me, "This looks almost like a scene from a horror movie."

"And the smell of the place makes it worse," he responded.

The pathologist glanced our way, and we became quiet as he began withdrawing the sheet from over the body. The subject of the autopsy was revealed as a thin, middle-aged male, waxen white, with bloodless lips, and closed, sunken eyes. The pathologist proceeded to open the abdominal cavity of the corpse with a scalpel. His commentary distracted us a little from the full impact of what was happening, as he explained he would work with the same precision and care as a surgeon performing an operation. He emphasised that anything we heard or saw was subject to the oath of confidentiality we had taken, and that we were bound to treat this patient with the same respect as any we met in a hospital. He removed each organ, examined, weighed and measured it, dictating his findings into a voice recorder as he worked.

After about half an hour, I found I was trying to suppress a feeling of queasiness. Out of the corner of my eye I noticed a female friend was looking rather pale, if not a little green. This took my mind off my own discomfort. Dimly, I heard the pathologist explain he was now moving to the nervous system and would need to examine the brain to rule out the possibility of a haemorrhage. The grinding noise of his electric bone saw cutting into the skull was interrupted by a crash as someone hit the floor. It was the big policeman.

The rest of the events and findings from that day are lost to me, but we had survived an important rite of passage which enabled us to subsequently attend and learn from postmortems as doctors, with less trepidation. Perhaps such experiences helped inure us to future contact with death. Days like these bound us together as a mutually supportive group in success and failure, a habit which benefited us well in later professional life. The friendships formed then, lasted a lifetime.

Science

I was less enthralled by several of the other biomedical sciences we studied. Sometimes our attitude was that we were almost marking time until we were qualified to attend hospitals and patients, when we would learn real Medicine. In part, this feeling was fostered by less inspirational lectures and lecturers, who couldn't compete with the anatomy showman. One of our teachers had an unfortunate, weary nasal delivery much mimicked by students. Another, treated more sympathetically, had an unfortunate speech impediment causing words to become intermittently trapped somewhere in her throat. Our embryology course was aborted when the lecturer became seriously ill, creating an unfortunate deficiency in my knowledge of foetal development for years. In biochemistry, I found the requirement to memorise and reproduce complex cellular metabolic pathways tedious. It was like being expected to memorise the internal circuitry of a mobile phone, before being allowed to use it.

The study of normal physiology was more interesting, being essential to understanding the diseases that are caused by systems malfunctioning - for example, when insulin production fails and diabetes results. For me, the related practical classes could not compete with anatomy dissection. Sometimes they lacked imagination. For instance, we once spent an afternoon measuring, half-hourly, our urine output, after drinking a couple of litres of water. Some students expressed the view that if beer had been substituted for water, it would have been a much more interesting experiment. In response, the laboratory supervisor pointed out that a practical class was hardly necessary to reproduce results already known to us from time spent in the Student's Union bar.

The simultaneous study of anatomy, biochemistry, physiology, histology (cellular anatomy), and embryology was demanding. It seemed we needed to spend much more time studying and attending courses than any of our friends taking degrees in engineering, pure science or the arts. This complex of science subjects did not kick in until our second year, when the workload began to isolate us socially from other undergraduates.

First year had been composed of a common cross-faculty science course which proved only a little more demanding than the advanced level studies at school, taken by most medical students. We became acclimatised to the freedom and challenges of university life, got to know our colleagues and had time to get involved in various student affairs, societies, politics, and sports. Above all, we began to mature and develop a broader outlook on life in general. The university was, in those days, primarily an educational establishment rather than a business.

Student life

In the late 1960s, Northern Ireland was as ever, a politically divided society. Like all children from the protestant community, I had attended a state school, as opposed to a catholic church school. After the UK Education Act of 1944, every child was guaranteed free schooling up to the age of 15 or 16. A similar Act was passed in 1947 by the local Stormont Parliament. Furthermore, there was a strong, grant-aided grammar school system locally, which was open to any child, irrespective of religion or background, providing they passed the qualifying 11-plus examination. Naively, I had expected to pass - not because of my mother's drive for her children to do well academically, but simply because my older brother had done so.

University had also come within the reach of many who, until then, had been denied such an opportunity. In 1962, when only 5 to 10% of the population went on to higher education, discretionary maintenance grants were introduced to cover tuition fees and living costs. When I enrolled, this amounted to £380 per annum, which may seem very little today, but the average annual working wage then was around £750, less than £15 per week. Many students supplemented their income by taking summer jobs. In my case, this involved traveling to a fruit and vegetable canning factory in Lincolnshire.

These educational opportunities meant that those of us starting our first year in medical school in 1965 came from a relatively diverse range of backgrounds and traditions, although the majority were still from middle class families. Nonetheless, many of us met and made friends with people from a different culture to our own, often for the first time. Initially, we would discreetly avoid discussing which schools we had attended, and thus avoid any perception that we might be trying to ascertain each other's religious or political allegiances. Generally, by the time such knowledge surfaced, it made little or no difference to the friendships we had formed. I found this quite liberating. Perhaps people who chose medicine as a career tended to be more tolerant? I became keen to get a clearer understanding of both republican and unionist politics, and of the contrasts between catholic and protestant traditions. I was already an admirer of Martin Luther King's non-violent battle for civil rights in America when I discovered the

9

Corrymeela Community. This was a movement being developed by a farsighted university chaplain, who was concerned by increasing sectarian tensions locally. He had been a prisoner of war in the 1940s, incarcerated in Dresden, and there had observed the devastating legacy of that conflict. Corrymeela brought students of various backgrounds, political and religious beliefs together to discuss our differences, and explore what we had in common. My contact with like-minded people there, working and hoping for a shared and peaceful future, confirmed in me a life-long belief in justice, equality and tolerance. More than 50 years on, that ethos remains as relevant and important as ever.

University terms seemed to pass twice as quickly as school terms, driven by the intense studying, and the demanding social life of dances, late night parties, and weekend sport. All too soon, the critical mid-course examinations were upon us - the final hurdle before embarking on clinical studies.

Fire, Fire!

On the evening before my final anatomy practical examination, I sat up late into the night revising the names and attachments of the many muscles in the body. Eventually, I held a long upper arm bone, the humerus, to which were connected the deltoid, biceps and triceps muscles. I had worked my way through all those in the legs, feet, spine, pelvis, hands and forearm. Many of the muscles were traditionally named in Latin, an added test of my memory power. Names like flexor pollicus longus, the muscle which bends the thumb to make a pincer with the opposed index finger, and enables humans to pick up objects, use tools, hold a pen and make notes. I was using the human skeleton which I owned to reinforce my knowledge of exactly where each muscle was attached to the relevant bone. By midnight, my brain was in overload, so I called it a day. I returned my dissection manuals and my anatomy atlas to the bookcase, glad to escape the impregnated smell of tissue preservative. I carefully packed the skeleton into its wooden box which I pushed under the bed, hoping I would never need it again. Then, after one last restorative cup of tea and a biscuit, I slid under the blankets in the front bedroom of my parent's terrace house.

Shortly, I would be facing the same formidable teacher I had met on that first day, this time in a practical and oral examination.

As I drifted toward sleep, I relaxed and smiled to myself, thinking of my mother's half-serious reaction when she first saw the skeleton I had brought home, and kept in the box in my room.

"At the last trump, when our Lord returns to resurrect his believers from down the ages," she wondered, "will a strange man appear from under your bed?"

"Don't worry," I reassured her with a laugh. "First of all, it's supposed to be a female skeleton and, furthermore, it is said to have come from India many years ago. So the original owner was probably a nonbeliever... or perhaps worshipped another God."

With this happy reminiscence, I slipped into a restless sleep.

Suddenly, I became aware of the unmistakable loud, urgent and repetitive ring-a-ding, ding-a-ling that was characteristic of fire engines and ambulances in the days before they were equipped with sirens, operating at 20 times the old-fashioned bell's decibel level. The noise seemed to be getting closer and closer. As I became more conscious, it dawned on me that the crescendo of ringing meant the din was no longer coming from the distant main road. This would not have been unusual, as there was a Fire Brigade Station about a mile away. No, it was undoubtedly approaching the small complex of streets in which we lived. Within a very short time, it became clear that the noise was approaching our house. Then it seemed to stop, almost outside.

Houses did not have double glazing at that time, so the noise from the street was easily audible in the stillness of the night. I could hear not only the firemen shouting, but also the sound of neighbours coming out of their houses to find out what exactly was happening, and calling out to each other. I arose wearily, pulled up the blackout window blind and stared out. I was soon joined by my parents, brother and sister. Shortly, my father donned some clothes, went downstairs and walked along the short garden path to talk with the neighbours. We waited impatiently for his return, and watched the extending ladder of the fire engine reaching up to the roof of a neighbouring house. Smoke and even a few flames could be seen issuing from the chimney. Some firemen were connecting a hosepipe to a fire hydrant, having removed a metal manhole cover on the pavement to locate the connection to the mains water supply. Another ran, carrying the other end of the hose, to the bottom of the ladder. He climbed expertly up to the roof, thrust the end of the hose into the chimney and called for the water to be turned on. Another hose was run from the fire engine through the front door of the burning house. Smoke and steam now belched from a downstairs window.

My father returned from his discussion with the small crowd which had gathered.

"Apparently Mr Kerr staggered home drunk a while ago. I bet he spent the evening at the Horseshoe Arms as usual."

Mr Kerr had been living on his own since his wife and children moved out a year earlier, so the house was probably freezing cold.

"One of the firemen reckons he couldn't get the fire to light, so he chucked some petrol on it. He managed to stagger next door and rap up the family there. They ran to the phone box and dialled 999. It seems everything in the living room was set alight. He's miraculously unharmed, apart from the alcohol. He has no actual burns except to his clothes. It's a real disaster for Andy - not only has he lost his family, but now he's lost his home."

I had only the slightest twinge of guilt as I prayed that the Fire Brigade would quench the fire and leave soon so that everyone, especially myself, could get back to bed, and perhaps get some essential sleep. At about 3 a.m., I swapped beds with my sister, who slept at the rear of our house. Four hours later, my alarm clock rang, and I was up again. My mother insisted I had a bowl of porridge and an Ulster Fry - bacon, eggs, potato and wheaten bread, to set me up for the exam.

Fortunately, despite the disrupted night, I must have performed reasonably well on those detailed questions about the skull and various bones. I found out a week later that I had passed the crucial MB examinations, enabling me to proceed to learn clinical medicine at the nearby major teaching hospital. What I did not realise at the time was that, eventually, as a junior doctor, performing under conditions of sleep deprivation would be a standard part of the job.

2. Meeting patients at last

Once we had satisfied the medical school, in year three, that we had a satisfactory grasp of the basic medical sciences, we were allowed to proceed to undertake clinical studies and training. This was the moment most of us had been waiting for, when we really became medical students involved in looking after and learning from patients. We were again divided alphabetically into groups of eight and allocated to medical or surgical wards in the major teaching hospitals near to the University. There was a quiet pride in gaining this position on the very lowest level of a ward clinical team. This consisted, from the top, of a consultant, then a senior registrar, a registrar, a senior house officer and a junior house officer. Senior registrars were generally next in line for consultant posts, while junior house officers had only just qualified as doctors. Conversely, we also held an unspoken, biased (and probably unfounded) perception that we were now at - or near - the top of the university undergraduate hierarchy.

From our experiences over succeeding years, most of us would learn humility and respect for people's feelings, beginning for me with the treatment of the young woman with a lump in her breast, as I will explain later.

Great relief

Once or more each week, the ward unit to which we were attached would accept all the new emergency admissions. Each new patient would be allocated a medical student. One of my early patients was an elderly gentleman who arrived in great discomfort, unable to pass urine. His bladder outlet had become obstructed by an enlarged prostate gland. The admitting surgeon cornered me, and asked if I knew how to pass a urinary catheter. I knew the technique but confessed I had, as yet, only catheterised one patient under supervision. Clearly harassed, he demanded, "Can you do it or not?"

"Yes, I think so," I stammered.

He rapidly introduced me to a staff nurse, informing me that she had assisted the procedure many times, and would keep me right if necessary. He hurried off, telling me to be as quick as I could, as our patient was clearly in

14

agony. He would, he reassured me, be back to check on me as soon as he had a free minute.

The nurse encouraged me to talk through each step of the procedure I planned, as we prepared the necessary equipment. She provided me with surgical gloves and antiseptic cleansing solutions. Fortunately, the catheter slipped easily through the penile urethra into the bladder and rapidly drained off over half a litre of urine before she advised me to clamp the tube and connect it to a drainage bag. The effect on the old man was dramatic. As I removed my surgical gloves he reached out his hand.

"Thank you, doctor, you have no idea what an enormous relief that is. I felt like I was going to die."

A tear spilled from his eye. I was discomforted by his gratitude - and that he had mistaken me for a doctor - but I recognised the vulnerability of an old person living alone with an embarrassing problem. I explained again, as I shook his hand, that I was actually a medical student. It was one of the first times I felt I was doing some practical good. Stepping outside the procedure room with me, the staff nurse grinned, happy to have helped, and punched me lightly on the arm.

"There you are, the next time you won't be needing my assistance," she said. And then she was gone.

I was to learn a lot from my nursing colleagues over the succeeding years.

The art of medicine: looking the part?

We had limited formal preparation for venturing into the wards but were each supplied with five, highly starched white coats and instructed we must always wear these in the hospital, with our name badge attached. These had our title, "Medical Student," printed in red across the top, making it clear to patients that we had not yet qualified as doctors. I suspect most would have had little difficulty reaching this conclusion, even without the badge. The coats were boiled, ironed and starched each week in the hospital laundry. The amount of starch incorporated into the cloth by the laundering process meant that considerable strength was required to fight one's arms down the sleeves. Initially, they were so stiff that our arm movements were, of necessity, rather robotic. We were expected to dress smartly: Men in shirts,

15

ties and sharply pressed trousers; women reasonably demurely - if not in slacks, then in dresses or skirts of a sensible length.

The white coats were to be spotless and buttoned up to ensure admission to the wards by the sister, and to reduce the risk of cross infection.

While there was little or no preparation for the actual face-to-face contact with patients, attention to the dress code was quite vigorous. I was once stopped in a corridor by the professor of surgery.

"Excuse me young man," he said. "Would you mind telling me your name?"

It was only when he produced a pen and wrote it on my coat that I realised my plastic name badge had fallen off. I cannot recollect him advising on any approach to dealing with ill patients. There was no communication skills course, no lessons or practice in bedside etiquette, merely an introductory lecture after which we were each provided with a thin blue booklet entitled, "Clinical History-Taking and Examination." It gave lists of questions relating to each body system. Respiratory - Do you have a cough? How long have you had the cough? Does coughing produce sputum? Is the sputum bloodstained? Do you have any pain in your chest? Is it difficult to breathe, and so on.

There were no clear instructions regarding how we might obtain consent from patients to have their history taken by a student, nor were we advised to explain that the person could refuse to be examined. It was generally assumed that patients in hospital accepted that students were part of the ward team. There were no suggestions as to how best we might win a patient's trust, learn about their hopes and fears or, indeed, how we might allay their worries. I had learnt from the elderly man with the urinary retention the importance of introducing myself and my status properly. I was beginning to grasp some of the art of practising medicine, a step beyond merely having an understanding of the underlying science. Our innate sense of appropriate behaviour was gradually refined by observing the more empathetic registrar tutors and senior consultants.

Now, I regularly encountered patients who were prepared to share personal, even intimate, details of their complaints and symptoms with me; who allowed me to examine them, and who, despite being ill, were often anxious to help me learn. In response, a desire for competence became the

16

driver of my studies. I was hungry to learn practical skills, to become proficient at diagnosis and to know appropriate treatments for the conditions which I encountered. While the range of diseases affecting the various body systems seemed vast, the challenge to learn all I could offered a unique sense of satisfaction from the hard work that demanded long hours of study. These were rewarding days.

Our responsibilities gradually increased as we gained experience and confidence. Initially on ward attachments called clinical clerkships, we obtained from patients details of their complaints, before examining them and making careful notes. We then presented our findings to doctors who corrected and expanded our work, teaching us to be more accurate, focused and competent. Eventually, as senior students, these so-called "clerk-ins" would be incorporated in the patient's clinical file.

Within a year, we were routinely taking blood samples, learning and performing basic procedures such as erecting intravenous infusions and gradually becoming more useful members of a ward team. In the Accident and Emergency Department we learnt how to suture wounds. Initially, if truth were told, we were employed to do so on drunk patients, thus relieving busy doctors to attend to more seriously ill individuals. I sutured a wound in a man who had arrived after a minor accident at a nearby metal foundry and became aware he was watching my work very carefully. I finished and cleaned away some blood before a nurse prepared to apply a dressing, when he suggested I might insert two or three more stitches. I could not see that they were necessary, but the nurse suggested it would do no harm, so I grudgingly complied. After the unusually grateful patient had left, I heard that the Foundry awarded compensation on the basis of the number of stitches required. Gaining skill at these practical procedures appealed to someone who came from a family of artisans, just as learning basic carpentry, as a child, from my grandfather had done. Back then, as I attempted to make toys from his wood offcuts, he had an encouraging adage for me: "The man who never made a mistake never made anything." I reflected that this did not really apply to the medical trade - where mistakes had potentially serious consequences. Today's students first practice taking medical histories from actors playing a pre-scripted role, and practical skills on mannequins, hopefully to the benefit of patients.

The art of medicine: respect

A young woman looked nervously at the group of medical students, new to the wards, who had gathered beside her bed. A nurse stepped forward to draw the curtains around it, at the request of the surgeon, who was conducting a teaching ward round. These rounds were the mainstay of the clinical teaching course. He had arrived with the eager entourage hanging on his every word. He was a tall, confident, commanding figure, possibly with a background in military service, leading his squad from bed to bed. His teaching method involved asking questions about the suggested diagnosis, the answers to which were often a mystery to most of us during these early weeks on our first surgical attachment. Having exposed our ignorance, he would impress us with his knowledge of the condition and his slick examination technique, all the while endeavouring to pass this on to us.

On this morning, he briefly smiled at the young woman, who was not much older than we were, and asked her in a kindly manner, when she had first noticed a lump in her breast.

We could barely hear her soft-spoken answer, as she explained it was when she was taking a bath around a month before. Turning away, he now questioned us.

"What other pertinent information would you like to know?"

"Is the lump painful?" someone suggested.

"Go ahead and ask Miss Jones," he instructed.

After further interrogation, during which the patient's replies became quieter as she shifted in the bed, he then turned to the staff nurse, and asked her, rather than the patient herself, to slip down the top of the young lady's nightdress.

As she did so, he turned his back on her and continued to talk to us with some authority on the subject of such lumps, and then selected one of the female students.

"My dear, would you demonstrate the correct method of breast examination and see if you can identify the lump which is worrying my young friend?"

The patient reluctantly lowered the bed sheet from under her chin. Her eyes were cast down and there was a marked flush on her cheeks. This spread to her neck and upper chest as she was examined. Feeling her discomfort, I felt compelled to look away, some of us even turning aside to avoid meeting her eyes. When my fellow student indicated that she had located the lump, the surgeon repeated the examination to confirm that she was correct. He spoke again to the patient in a kindly voice.

"I am almost certain that this little lump is benign, and not anything serious to worry about, but as we discussed, to be certain I need to carry out a biopsy or remove it." He smiled reassuringly.

He then instructed another student, a male this time, to palpate the lump. Meanwhile he emphasised to the group that it was imperative for all doctors to be able to identify the smallest lump in the female breast, because of the risk of malignancy.

It suddenly struck me that our teacher was probably intending that other students, perhaps all of us, would examine the patient. Indeed, another student was soon enlisted. A few moments later the staff nurse, whose temporary absence I had not noticed, reappeared with the ward sister. She greeted the surgeon with deference, but stepped forward to draw up the patient's nightdress.

"Good morning sir, I believe you were anxious for the students to see our lady with the jaundice?" she suggested politely. "She is just two beds along and quite happy to see the medical students."

He looked at the sister for a few seconds and then said, "Of course, I was forgetting about Mrs. McManus, a lovely lady. I'll come with you and leave the staff nurse to help Miss Jones get sorted."

With that, the sister ushered the group along the ward to the next patient. We had no hesitation in following her lead. As we filed out from behind the curtains, I was sure I saw a few tears on the girl's cheeks as she tried to keep her composure. Still reluctant to make eye contact, I rejected any thought of thanking her. That evening, I wondered if anyone had thought to apologise to the patient for her unfortunate experience. I realised words from a male student would undoubtedly have embarrassed her further. I hoped she would not be found to have a malignant tumour.

Several days later, I encountered the nurse who had chaperoned the ward round, in the hospital corridor. I asked her if she knew the outcome of the patient's operation. She looked at me for a few seconds, probably not remembering me, or perhaps gauging how much she should say. I felt uncomfortable again as she hesitated.

"Actually, she was going to sign herself out after you students left, but sister spoke with her and she went to theatre as planned."

The nurse's tone indicated she did not blame the girl.

"Most importantly, nothing sinister was found in the tissue sample."

With that she hurried off.

The judge

During the three years of clinical training, time was spent in each sub-specialty, with two long spells in each of general surgery and general medicine. Running in parallel were lecture-based courses in the relevant pharmacology, microbiology and pathology of disease.

On a winter medical "take in" day, there might be 20 or 30 admissions, far in excess of the number of beds available in any general ward, and so empty beds in other units were requisitioned. The number of hospital beds has steadily declined since then, so that the term "trolly waits" has been coined for those unfortunate enough to require inpatient treatment when, as is often the case, a bed cannot be found.

Consultant staff rarely saw those admitted overnight by their registrars, so they started a long "pick up" round early next morning. This sometimes lasted into the afternoon. Before it started, we students were tasked with taking blood samples for any laboratory tests which had been ordered overnight. While some senior doctors took the attitude that consultants were there to be consulted, the specialist to whom I was attached reviewed every patient and their treatment after admission. He made a point of speaking to each one personally and frequently, as well as meeting anxious relatives. I watched and learned from him as he listened carefully, responded clearly and authoritatively, noting the reassurance he provided.

Respiratory complaints, heart disease and strokes were common diagnoses. Heart attacks were aggressively managed, strokes less so. This was an era when the absence of scanning technology made it difficult to differentiate between haemorrhage (bleeding into the brain) and ischaemia (where the circulation is blocked) as the underlying cause of a stroke.

It seems bizarre today that smoking was allowed in the wards, not to mention that the worthy volunteers of the Ladies' League brought round a trolly of various items for sale each day, including cigarettes as well as toiletries, magazines, and sweets.

On one pick up round, an elderly gentleman, Mr Andrews, who had lost most of his power of speech and the strength of his right side from a stroke, listened carefully as our teacher explained his condition to his wife and the students. He became distressed and finally managed one word.

"Home!"

"I'm afraid you are not quite ready for home just yet," the consultant explained, "but perhaps in a day or two."

The call was repeated as we proceeded from bed to bed. "Home!"

A few days later Mr Andrews had recovered a little more speech and on spotting the consultant in the ward again, with considerable effort, called out, "Home... now!"

Once more it was firmly, but kindly, pointed out that he needed speech therapy, physiotherapy and his blood pressure controlled. Mr Andrews shook his head. "Home! Home!"

"I'll be the judge of when you are ready," was the reply.

Over the next two weeks every time the professor appeared, a cry of "The Judge! The Judge!"now pursued him.

We took to referring to Mr Andrews himself as "The Judge" as we watched his progress. At last, he recovered sufficiently to be able to leave the ward, leaning on a stick. He shook hands with our boss, using his right hand with difficulty.

"The Judge," he said, clearly meaning himself, as he indicated his chest with his good hand, before moving determinedly on.

21

"Manifestly a fighter, I have no doubt he will continue to improve," remarked the chief judge.

Good communication is not always easy.

In the country of the blind

The course in ophthalmology was short, so there was only a cursory demonstration in the use of the ophthalmoscope for examining the various structures and chambers of the eye. The consultant leading this introductory teaching session then left us to practice on each other, using instruments that we had each been required to purchase at considerable expense. A valuable investment, as it turned out. I still have mine, which continues to work efficiently. On that first day, most of us had difficulty focusing on the corneal surface, the lens behind, or the retina, with its blood vessels and the central optic nerve at the back of the eye.

In the next session we were led into a darkened room (to aid dilatation of the pupil) in which were seated several volunteer patients. Our teacher selected a victim from our student group and asked if he had been practising with the ophthalmoscope. He received a muttered affirmative response.

"So, if I ask you to have a look at one of these patients, who have come along to help with your education, can I assume you are reasonably competent with the instrument?"

Not wishing to embarrass himself in front of his teacher, colleagues, nurses and the patients, the victim agreed he had met with some success examining his friend's eyes.

"Excellent," said the eminent specialist. "I wonder if you would look at my friend's left eye and tell me what you think his problem might be."

Turning to the elderly gentleman he asked, "It's true that, essentially, you can see nothing with your left eye?"

The gentleman agreed and the student placed his ophthalmoscope close to his own right eye and focused on Mr Elder's left one. After several minutes, it became obvious that he was having considerable difficulty, as he repeatedly shifted position and altered the settings on the instrument. When the ophthalmologist began to drum his fingers on his desk, he stopped and stepped back. We looked on sympathetically as the lights in the room were switched on.

"Well, young man, what can you tell us?"

"Not very much," was the reply. "I am sorry, but I couldn't focus on any of the structures of the eye at all."

"Well, well, well. Perhaps the patient can enlighten us all to the nature of his problem?"

He turned to the patient, tilted his head and raised a quizzical eyebrow. At this, the patient, whom we later realised had been primed to give a performance, raised his hands to his face and used his index fingers to pop out a prosthetic "glass" eye, which he proffered to the shocked student. Mr Elder, the doctor, and a couple of nurses who were in on the act laughed, enjoying his discomfort. Most of the student group also thought the pantomime was quite funny. We were to become immune to education by humiliation.

We regularly critiqued the attitudes and performance of our teachers, those of us with no family medical background perhaps being more judgemental. Subconsciously, we were looking for role models for the sort of doctor we wished to become. While I developed an enormous respect for the majority of physicians and surgeons I encountered in my undergraduate training, some of those who fell short of my idealism also left a lasting impression.

On another attachment, on this occasion to a peripheral hospital, a doctor with what might be described as a public-school accent, despite his local origins and education, was examining a man's respiratory tract. He had been admitted with an exacerbation of a chronic chest condition. The doctor's first action was to place a forefinger on the patient's chin and turn his head away, without explanation. Later, moving along the ward, he asked if we appreciated the importance of this preliminary move. Someone suggested that this was in order to evaluate the jugular vein pressure which, if visibly raised in the neck, is a sign of heart failure. Others agreed.

"No, it was so that when I bent down to listen to his chest with my stethoscope, he would not breathe on me," he explained.

Someone asked if perhaps he suspected Tuberculosis.

"No, no! Some of these chaps have terrible halitosis and, indeed, rather poor hygiene in general."

Cringing, I glanced back to see if we were within hearing distance of the patient. My respect for this teacher was similar to his, towards his patient.

On board the cardiac ambulance

The ambulance, also known as The Heart Cart, raced through the rush hour traffic, siren wailing, then halted beside a small crowd which had gathered opposite the City Hall. We leapt out of the rear door. People stepped aside and we could see a man lying prostrate on the pavement. The young woman kneeling beside him looked up with relief, quickly explained that she was a nurse and that the man had collapsed on his way home from work and was complaining of severe chest pain. His lips had a blueish tinge and he was breathing with difficulty as he attempted to speak. The doctor and specialist nurse on our team immediately took over. My role, as a now senior medical student, was mainly to carry equipment and, of course, to learn.

A spell on attachment to the cardiac unit in the Royal Victoria Hospital gave a unique opportunity to be at the forefront of medical innovation. Professor Pantridge, a taciturn man with a forceful personality led the team, and locally, had a legendary status. He had been awarded the Military Cross during the Second World War, then, in civilian life, had successfully advocated the cardiopulmonary resuscitation technique known today as CPR. Since this has become such standard practice, it is difficult to imagine there was a time when it was not so. Today, it is taught in virtually every secondary school and workplace.

The development of the rapid response cardiac ambulance service resulted from his realisation that death following a coronary heart attack was often due to the heart's pumping rhythm becoming erratic and inefficient. This abnormal rhythm, known as ventricular fibrillation, inevitably led to total cardiac arrest and death. He recognised there was a short window of time when the heart could be electronically shocked back into a normal rhythm and function. The equipment to do this, a defibrillator, was initially only available in hospitals until Pantridge developed a relatively portable version that could be carried in an ambulance to the patient.

On this, one of my first experiences of such a critical situation outside hospital, it became clear that the man's circulation was so compromised that it was difficult to place anything other than a very fine needle in a vein to deliver essential medication and pain relief.

"Do you know how to perform a cutdown into the large saphenous leg vein?" demanded the cardiac registrar. I confirmed that I had done so a couple of times. As he examined the cardiograph trace, he urged, "See if you can manage it again. We need to get good vascular access to deliver drugs."

Almost immediately the nurse had the sterile "cutdown" pack open beside me on the pavement. I pulled on surgical gloves and picked up a scalpel. I made a tiny incision above the ankle, where my anatomy training had taught me the vein would be situated, even if it was not visible. Minutes later, a cannula was in the exposed vessel and medication was being infused to stabilise the heart and alleviate pain. As I concentrated on inserting a stitch into the skin to hold the line in place, I became aware that a crowd was still around us. Then I heard a broad Belfast accent announcing,

"My God they're actually operatin' on him in the middle of the street!''

On another occasion, as we drew up at the address to which we had been called, we realised it was that of a Funeral Parlour. We dashed in, wondering what to expect. To our relief the patient was not lying in a coffin but on the office floor. The undertaker fortunately survived and avoided becoming a client on his own premises.

Sunday in Northern Ireland was then a very quiet day, with shops, pubs and cinemas closed, while Church attendance was high. Unusually on this traditional day of rest, we attended two emergencies. The morning call was to a Plymouth Brethren Meeting Hall. Inside, the Believers sat in rows around the four sides of a table on which were set out the communion bread and wine. An elderly gentleman had been laid down on the floor beside it, surrounded by the silent congregation. He was distressed and short of breath. Loosening his waistcoat, shirt and tie, I set about attaching ECG leads to his chest, while the team doctor examined him and our nurse spoke softly and reassuringly in the hushed atmosphere. The tracing showed an erratic heart rhythm. As an intravenous cannula was prepared, one of the worshippers rose to his feet.

"Brothers and sisters," he said in a solemn tone, "let us quietly pray that our Lord guides the hands of these young doctors and nurses today and restores our brother to full health." He sat down and heads were bowed. "No pressure then," I thought, as the registrar palpated the patient's arm to locate a vein. Shortly the patient was stable, with an improved blood pressure, no longer in pain and we were ready to transport him off to hospital.

Later in the afternoon, we arrived at a house in the south of the city. We were ushered into a bedroom by the wife of a man suffering severe chest pain. It had eased a little, but he was clearly frightened, very pale, and relieved to see us. He was quickly administered an injection to alleviate his pain and began to look less distressed. As we set about assessing his condition further, checking his blood pressure and obtaining an ECG trace, the team doctor inquired what our patient had been doing when the pain came on. The man hesitated, then said he had been in bed. Our doctor that day was one of those intellectually brilliant people who lacked a little social awareness.

"So," he said, making a note, "you were having a bit of a rest, not doing anything strenuous at all?" Our patient looked away for a moment, and made no response. His wife, looking a little embarrassed, interjected.

"We were both in bed." She explained.

He looked at her quizzically.

The nurse leaned over and spoke inaudibly in the doctor's ear. He became briefly flustered before regaining a professional air and examining the cardiogram trace. I noticed he had blushed, generally an uncommon reaction in members of the medical profession.

He reassured the couple that, although there was evidence of a mild heart attack, he felt there was no immediate danger but would bring the husband into hospital for further tests and observation.

As students, we sometimes received very personal information. Observing this sort of exchange emphasised to me the need to treat such confidences with delicacy.

Any life and death situation demands a rapid reaction and of course divine help is always welcome. Stabilising a critically ill individual and getting them to a place of safety is the priority. After a month on this team, often only as an observer, I remembered forever the importance of suppressing personal feelings of panic in order to, at least, appear calm and focus on what needs to be done in an emergency. I was developing an altered, professional, adrenalin-driven response when faced with the approaching spectre of death; fear and fight. Fear that we might fail to save the patient, combined with a determination to fight with our utmost ability to succeed. Flight is not an option. The learned reflex was to move towards rather than away from the crisis. The heightened tension, compounded by the short time we had to respond, was compensated for by the thrill of delivering a patient to the intensive care ward alive. Failure was always emotional and depressing and, for those in the key roles, exhausting. I came to recognise that the chances of survival from a cardiac arrest outside a hospital environment was only 15%. Even in hospitals, the figure only grew to 40%. It has often been said that the best place of all to suffer a cardiac arrest is in a TV drama, where survival rates are estimated to be up to 75%.

Perhaps these figures require updating now that there are defibrillators in workplaces, sports facilities, and even shops across the country. All part of Professor Pantridge's legacy, leading tothe development of today's rapid-response, highly skilled, Paramedic ambulance crews.

A child is born

On a winter afternoon, I spent an hour or more in the labour ward talking with Mrs. Keegan, a friendly woman in her mid-thirties. I had been given the responsibility of monitoring her progress. She told me she already had five children and was married to a handsome, hard-working builder. He was due to arrive on the ward shortly, after he had farmed out their children to relatives or neighbours. I learned that she came from a family of eight and had always wanted a big family herself. Sitting up in bed, she told me happily about her previous labours and of some of her two older sons' escapades. As time went by, she intermittently paused and reached for the Entonox gas and air device. This 50/50 mixture of nitrous oxide and oxygen takes the edge off labour pains. It is also known as laughing gas, although not many women

27

laugh much during labour. After four or five deep breaths from the mask, she chatted on.

Medical students were expected to deliver 20 babies to qualify for the degree of Bachelor of the Art of Obstetrics (BAO). I was allocated to the main maternity hospital for the residential course which, despite rather substandard accommodation, was much sought after because of the experience it guaranteed. We competed for deliveries against student midwives, who were also expected to attend a large quota of births. The labour ward and the allocation of patients was overseen by the Sister. If she deemed a medical student was tardy in arriving after she activated their radio bleep, the delivery quickly passed to one of her student midwives. Sister was proud of her early training and experience in the Queen Alexandra's Army Nursing Corp, and her ward was run with military precision, with medical students in the role of raw recruits. We would, of course, rush to the ward from whatever we were doing, whether attending lectures, ward rounds, studying, or even sleeping in bed upstairs. It was extremely irritating to arrive to find a mother well advanced in labour, with a student midwife already present under the protective eye of the Sister. To openly challenge this bias generally meant we were unlikely to receive a call again any time soon. It was a matter of some discussion that the midwifery students inevitably seemed to be ahead of us in reaching their target number of deliveries.

It is difficult to describe the impact of seeing a baby being born for the first time. It brought a new meaning to phrases like "the miracle of birth" and "the gift of a child". Along with the awe, came the sobering realisation that I would soon be expected to deliver someone's precious baby. Gradually, we moved from being enthralled observers, to assisting experienced midwives and then, under close supervision, performing a delivery. I doubt if I fully appreciated the gift mothers gave in allowing me to be involved, until I was present at one of my own children's births and my wife, Anne, showed the same generosity to a student midwife.

Before the afternoon I spent with Mrs. Keegan, I had delivered several babies and was confident enough checking the baby's heartbeat through a funnel-shaped foetal stethoscope pressed against Mrs. Keegan's protuberant tummy as the contractions built. Ultrasound monitors were not yet in common use. The senior midwife regularly joined us to check the degree of cervical dilation.

At some point, Mrs. Keegan took a longer than usual go at the Entonox, then said to me, "I think I need to push."

"Okay," I said, "I'll just let Sister know what's happening. You just take big, deep breaths and try to relax until the next contraction. You've done all this before, as you've been telling me."

I gave her my most encouraging smile. Outside her room, there was no one in sight.

"Hello!" I called anxiously, "Is there a midwife free?"

Getting no response, I returned to join my patient, and discreetly pressed the emergency call button.

After the next long suck on the gas and air, my patient announced in no uncertain terms, "I really need to push NOW!" and adjusted her position appropriately.

Washing my hands for possibly the tenth time, I pulled on a fresh pair of gloves and examined her. I could already see the baby had dark hair and was ready to make a full appearance. I gently touched the surface of the head and advised, "Try not to push too hard, take lots of short breaths and, as you pant, the baby will come gently."

At that, Mrs. Keegan produced a noise from the back of her throat, as she gave a mighty push.

As the baby appeared at speed, I was thinking, "Where in God's name is Sister?"

I carefully supported the baby's head as he slid out into my hands. Suddenly there was someone beside me wrapping the baby in a soft clean towel and saying, in a warm congratulatory tone, "Beautifully done," not to me, but to the baby's mother, who had indeed performed superbly. With slightly shaking hands, I applied the umbilical clamp and cut the cord as the baby let everyone know he had entered the world. Sister placed him on his mum's chest and turned to me with a mischievous grin as she said, "No

29

problems there, then, doctor? Quick work, eh? Don't forget to write everything up in the notes."

With that, she left.

A little later, with the placenta delivered, and mum and the ward tidied up, the father arrived. A cup of tea had been ordered and was on its way.

"Would you like to hold the wee lad?" he asked, after he had nursed his new son long enough.

Taking the baby, I looked down at him in my arms, no doubt with a silly, satisfied smile on my face, as if I had really played all that significant a role in events. The pleased and proud mother spoke up, "If you don't mind me asking, doctor, what is your first name?"

"Why, not at all," I said, "it's Maurice."

She looked at her husband.

"That's a lovely name" she said, diplomatically. "I think this one's going to be called after his uncle Gerry."

"Aye, he looks like a Gerry alright," said his dad.

Although the midwives did most of the delivering and nursing care of the babies and mothers, the consultant obstetricians were almost treated with reverence. They were expected to save the day, the mother and the baby, should dangerous situations develop. Strangely, this was a male dominated profession. There were no female obstetricians in what was otherwise a woman's world. The consultants paid special attention to women with more complex medical problems - mothers with heart disease, hypertension, diabetes or toxaemia, conditions which might affect the pregnancy or inhibit the baby's growth while still in the womb. They also concentrated on mothers who had previously experienced problems in pregnancy and, of course, those who paid to see them privately. There was even a special ward for such paying patients on the top floor of the hospital. Students did not venture there.

Neonatal care

The neonatal unit for premature and ill newborns had an air of controlled tension and proficiency. The midwives there struck me as having the confidence to cope with almost any situation; people from whom a lot could be learnt. For some, their work seemed to almost be their entire life. Their quiet efficiency among the incubators and bleeping monitors, as they nursed their tiny charges, spurred on my developing interest in paediatrics. Medically, the ward seemed to be run by a slightly maverick senior registrar, who was determined it should become one of the top units in the country. His long hair and drooped moustache marked him out from the traditional three-piece suit obstetric brigade. To me, he was the new generation. The measured humour and sound clinical ability shared by him and the neonatal sisters lightened the demanding work of caring for these precarious survivors, and the stressed, anxious parents. On at least one occasion, I observed the calming effect of the registrar's arrival, taking control of a situation almost before he initiated any action. Generous by nature, he was easily persuaded to give extra tutorials to the few of us who found his approach an inspiration. It was my pleasure, years later, to become his junior colleague.

This was a different world to adult medicine. Here, I watched tiny individuals, who might fit into the palms of my hands, fighting for their lives. Several babies were only in the unit because of their small size, with no other specific problems. All were under 2.5Kg (five and a half pounds) Some were small because they had been born early, before 36 weeks of pregnancy; these were the premature babies. Others were small because the placenta had become inefficient at providing adequate nutrition for some time before delivery. They were classified as "small for dates" babies. The two groups were faced with slightly different hazards in their early weeks. Topping the list for those born prematurely, were breathing problems. Those in either category may have required resuscitation at birth.

In the final few weeks of gestation, the developing lungs start to make a substance called surfactant. This reduces the surface tension in the tiny terminal air sacs, enhancing inflation. Anyone who has blown up balloons for a party knows the maximum effort is in getting the balloon open the first few centimetres. Without surfactant, the babies 'respiratory air sacs collapse back down with each expiration. A maximum inspiratory effort is then needed to re-inflate them with each breath and allow the life-giving oxygen to be transferred into the pulmonary blood stream. Supplemental oxygen helps, but some will need artificial ventilation, before they become exhausted.

Some babies were admitted with heart defects or other problems requiring surgery. A few had severe jaundice, which can harm the immature brain. These babies generally had a rhesus blood group incompatible with that of their mother. One afternoon, I stayed behind to watch a baby having its blood exchanged with that of a suitable donor to prevent further jaundice developing. Suddenly, a crash call for a paediatrician came from the labour ward. Rushing past, he called asking if I would like to join him. I quickly abandoned observing the exchange transfusion and ran with him to the delivery suite.

A mother was already being anaesthetised in the operating theatre for an emergency caesarean section. As her baby entered the birth canal, the umbilical cord had appeared first. There was an immediate danger of the advancing head crushing the prolapsed cord, and cutting off the blood and oxygen supply from the placenta to the unborn child. The baby needed to be rapidly delivered from above. A prolapsed chord is always an obstetric emergency.

The obstetrician was gowned and gloved. He identified me as an extra pair of hands.

"You," he said in a voice which broached no dissent, "quickly scrub and pull on a pair of sterile gloves. Get under the operating table and try to hold the baby's head back as best you can."

Without thought, I did as instructed, and cautiously probed two or maybe three fingers into the birth canal. I immediately felt the head and, avoiding the soft fontanelle, pushed tentatively upwards. I could feel the power of a uterine contraction beginning to bend my fingers, then suddenly the head was gone. I crawled out on my hands and knees from under the sterile drapes, feeling rather foolish. The paediatrician was holding a mask over the baby's mouth and nose, gently squeezing oxygen into her lungs. He had a stethoscope in his ears, while a nurse held the other end against the newborn's chest. Another was attaching ECG leads there. A smile appeared on the paediatrician's face. He withdrew the mask and we all heard a weak cry, which rapidly built to drown out the sound of the cardiac monitor. I don't think anyone actually cheered, but I certainly felt like it. The obstetrician was meticulously repairing his incision. I waited in the background to see the little girl in her mother's arms, admiring and maybe even envying the paediatrician a little, as he handed her over.

The social drinker

The senior surgical ward attachment in the final year involved clerking in twenty patients and producing a duplicate copy of their clinical case histories with a commentary on their presentation, diagnosis, treatment and prognosis. These were then scrutinised and marked by a supervising consultant. I was determined to collect as many unusual and informative cases as possible.

On a Thursday evening, when all emergency admissions were directed to our ward, the staff nurse let me know that a patient who was vomiting blood had been admitted. I hurried to the unit, quickly read his file and, drawing curtains around his bed to afford some privacy, introduced myself. Mr Jones, a fifty-six year old shipyard worker, shook my hand as firmly as he could, although I detected a slight tremor in his grip. In his left arm there was already an intravenous saline infusion running. He told me that, although he felt very unwell and sick, he was in no great pain. I recognised he was not the sort of man given to complaining unnecessarily. He volunteered that he had been diagnosed with liver cirrhosis, after being investigated at an outpatient clinic.

"Can cirrhosis make you vomit blood?" he asked anxiously.

I confirmed that it was not only possible but thought to be the most likely cause in his case. I explained that while we would replace the blood he had already lost, it would be equally important to arrest further internal bleeding.

I knew from the notes in his file that the possibility of surgical intervention had already been explained to him in the Emergency Department. They had arranged an urgent admission and sent a blood sample for biochemical analysis, blood group confirmation and cross matching against several units of donated blood.

I decided it was not the time to reiterate that his liver had been gradually damaged over years by alcohol consumption. Much of his hepatic tissue had undoubtedly been replaced by scar tissue which was now preventing blood filtering through the organ normally. Instead, the blood flow was being diverted into adjacent vessels in the lining of the oesophagus and stomach where, under high pressure, they had become engorged. That night, some of the swollen veins had burst, causing a life-threatening haemorrhage. I tried to reassure him as best I could, although I knew his situation was precarious. I explained that my consultant would be along immediately and would be best able to answer his questions. The results of blood tests would also be through shortly. The surgeon would determine what treatment was necessary to arrest any further blood loss. I emphasised that he was a top gastroenterologist, and that Mr Jones would be in expert hands. I tried to be positive but not say too much.

"The thing is," he said, "I'm not a big drinker. A lot of my mates drink far more than me. I've tried to cut my drinking down. I only take one or two at the weekends now, just to be sociable"

I nodded sympathetically, concealing my cynicism.

I tried to steer the conversation away from his alcohol habit, to establish if he had any other medical conditions and, importantly, any symptoms of heart disease.

He suddenly interrupted me mid-sentence and gasped, "Doctor, I think I'm going to be sick again."

Quickly, I stepped out from behind the curtains, looking urgently for a nurse. There was no-one in sight. I heard the man retching behind me, snatched a stainless steel basin and gave it to him. He looked desperately pale and much more unwell than just a minute before. His eyes were almost bulging as he tried to suppress his heaving stomach. His teeth were clamped together behind grimacing lips. I put an arm around him and held his shoulders as, abandoning any attempt to hold back, he leant forward and effortlessly almost filled the bowl with what looked like pure blood. As he fell back onto his pillows looking relieved, I was shocked by what I had seen at close quarters - and by a smell I was unlikely to ever forget. Keep calm, I told myself and pressed the emergency call button.

I was almost immediately joined by a nurse, then a second, and then the senior surgeon on the unit, in quick succession. The surgeon rapidly examined Mr Jones, as one of the nurses checked his blood pressure. He looked at me.

"The BP has fallen. The pulse is fast but weak. What are you going to do?" he asked in his slightly nasal staccato voice. Already rattled by the dramatic turn of events, I stuttered, "I'm just the medical student here."

I was afraid that he thought I was the house surgeon. His eyes narrowed.

"What are *we* going to do?" he demanded again.

"Quickly give him a unit of O negative blood?" I hazarded, knowing it could be given in emergencies to patients of any blood group. He confirmed this was on its way and turning to Mr Jones, he grasped his upper arm firmly. "We need to get you to the theatre to stop this bleeding. You are losing blood from veins in your stomach and the gullet, which we call the Oesophagus. When we have you asleep, I will inject them with something to clot the blood and seal the vessels. This young man and the nurse will give you an infusion of a drug through the drip to shut down the bleeding vessels which will stop, or at least slow, the bleeding temporarily, while we get everything ready."

He beckoned to the senior nurse and me as he stepped into the ward and wrote rapidly in the drug sheet.

"Give him twenty units of Pitressin Tannate in two hundred millilitres of normal saline, run in over twenty minutes, then the first unit of blood." He walked briskly away, heading for the operating theatre.

Still shocked by the speed of events, I asked the nurse, "Can we organise this?"

"Yes, I've done it before. Let's hope it works and we don't have to pass a balloon tube down his throat and inflate it to compress the swollen varicose vessels there. That's the next option. It's horrible for the patient. Oh, and the registrar just called to say he was on his way."

I gave thanks for this news.

We prepared the infusion as quickly as we could and rejoined the patient.

"This is the injection the surgeon has ordered," we explained. "It can make you feel worse for a short time and may give you abdominal cramps, as it constricts all the vessels near your stomach, but it is worth it."

As we started the infusion, we didn't add what we were thinking, "And it just might save your life."

A short time later, the registrar and an anaesthetist arrived to review the patient's condition. I joined them and was horrified by Mr Jones' appearance. He was deathly white. I had a moment's fear that we had got the dose wrong. The registrar looked at the chart recording Mr Jones's vital signs, and I was relieved to hear him tell the patient that his blood pressure was holding steady, the Pitressin injection had worked and they were ready for theatre.

A hand was raised weakly in acknowledgment.

It was the first time I had been so closely involved in such a haemorrhagic emergency. I wanted to see it through and accompanied my patient to the operating theatre. I watched the consultant surgeon expertly deal with the bleeding vessels. I felt a great sense of relief as he confirmed he had got all the bleeders injected and arrested the haemorrhage.

It had been an emotional rollercoaster of a night, frightening but ultimately satisfying. The fear of losing a patient can be like ice in your veins. I reflected that it was forty times worse for the patient.

This crisis was over but I knew it might recur, as blood still was unable to freely pass through Mr Jones's diseased liver. Major vascular surgery might address this. It would involve moving the portal vein, which carries most of the blood to the liver in order to divert the flow. Instead, it could be connected to the main vessel returning blood to the heart, the Vena Cava, thus by-passing the liver. Sadly, I was aware these measures would only buy some time and temporarily prolong his life.

It is the only case of the 20 that I clerked and submitted that I still remember.

Meanwhile, unknown to me and most of the world, Professor Roy Calne in Addenbrooke's hospital in Cambridge was developing the technique of liver transplantation. In years to come, this would bring hope of a return to normal life for patients with advanced liver disease.

A dramatic initiation

A toddler, just over a year old, is sitting on his mother's knee. Suddenly he makes a strange cry and seems to struggle to breathe. His lips turn bluish and his eyes roll up, the pupils barely visible. His left arm is jerking, then all four limbs shake. A nurse rushes over, picks him up and lays him on his side. An oxygen mask is held over his face. His skin is hot to touch. A doctor arrives and quickly assesses the seizure. She asks me to hold the child's wrist and hand steady, in a tight grip. I am almost shaking myself. With difficulty, she inserts a fine cannula into a vein in the back of the hand and slowly injects an anticonvulsant. The fit gradually subsides, his colour returns to normal. The little boy seems to be sleeping now. I have been horrified by the speed of development of (what appeared to me to be) a life-threatening event. In a few minutes, he opens his eyes, sees his mum and starts to cry. She takes him in her arms, whispers in his ear and rocks him gently.

This was one of my first days observing in the Children's Accident and Emergency Department, where I had once been a patient myself, aged eleven, after flying over the handlebars of my bicycle and splitting open my head.

A gentle touch

The Head of Paediatrics looked like a benign grandfather, with his white hair curling over his ears at the sides and thinning strands straggling over the top, although he was probably only in his fifties when I first met him. He always seemed to have a kindly smile and understanding concern when talking to parents. When he bent down to talk with small children, there was often a twinkle in his eye. His attitude to his students was one of encouragement, even when we were being grilled in formal examinations, although we suspected a certain leniency towards the female students. His specialty was gastroenterology and, in particular, excessive vomiting in babies. He was a world expert in infant Gastro Oesophageal Reflux and Congenital Hiatal Hernia - which he called Partial Thoracic Stomach. There was a generally accepted view that babies spewed and regurgitated small mouthfuls of milk as normal behaviour. He identified those in whom the habit was excessive, resulting in poor weight gain and distress - for parents and infants alike.

His research had demonstrated that this was frequently due to a minor anatomical problem, where the sphincter muscle at the stomach entry was displaced upwards to sit above the diaphragm. This meant it failed to close and stop milk and acid being regurgitated. He advocated nursing the babies in an upright position after a feed, in a device not unlike a modern infant car seat.

I recall sitting in his clinic, where mothers would enter with not only a baby but a towelling nappy or cloth draped over their shoulder to protect their clothes. At last, they would realise, they had found someone who appreciated the magnitude of their problem, as he listened sympathetically to their fear that the baby must have some awful illness. At least one told of how their homes smelled of either baby vomit or disinfectant. Some would confess tearfully that they were at their wit's end and felt like total failures.

He would explain emphatically that the poor weight gain was not due to some lack of mothering skill. He reassured them that he knew of at least fifty babies with the same problem, all of whom had done well following his advice and treatment. By the end of the consultation, a plan would be in place and his tendency to lay an encouraging hand on a mother or father's shoulder as they left, seemed to have an added positive placebo effect. Perhaps only subconsciously, at first, I registered that this might be the sort of doctor I aspired to be.

Today Reflux is more easily and successfully treated with the help of drugs that reduce gastric acid production.

Rebecca

I came to know Becky, the child who welcomed me on my first day as a student, a lot better during my stint in the children's ward. She was almost a member of the staff, joining us in the office, on ward rounds and coffee breaks.

Her family were desperate to get her home but managing her airway outside the hospital was considered to be too risky for such a young child.

She was an affectionate little girl, who was usually happy, except on a rare occasion when things did not go her way. Like many toddlers, she could throw a temper tantrum. It was hard not to capitulate to the demands of a distressed child crying silent tears. If the situation was not quickly

38

resolved, there was a danger it might escalate out of control. When Rebecca had exhausted every other option to get exactly what she wanted, she had been known, in a rage, to pull out her "trachy" tube with a flick of a little finger. This ultimate act of defiance demanded immediate and frantic action to cut the attached tapes in order to release and reinsert the plastic airway. Not only could she not get enough air into her lungs with it removed but there was a more serious risk that the skin opening might collapse and close over completely. It was a matter of debate as to whether such an emergency took more out of Rebecca or out of the shaken doctors and nurses who rushed to deal with the situation. Of course, once the drama was over, Rebecca would, contrite, sobbing, and frightened, revert to her normal vivacious and more rational self. Everyone would be offering to hug and cuddle her, to make her feel better. She would quickly bounce back and, with the drama forgotten, declined to bear a grudge. This little girl, forced to live in a totally abnormal environment, had an innate ability to adapt, to cope and even to fight the regime.

The longer she remained in hospital, the less control her parents felt they had over her future, which depended on her doctors finding a solution to her problem. This was not long after the days when parents could only visit wards for an hour on Saturdays and Sundays. By the 1960s, a daily visiting time had been introduced. As students, we heard worries that Becky was becoming institutionalised. She seemed to accept that the hospital was her home. It was almost as if Rebecca belonged to the hospital, rather than her mum and dad. I could understand that this might have long term effects on her future behaviour and relationships. Personally, I was impressed that she still had plenty of spirit. Her parent's needs and fears were not something I remember being discussed with us as students, although we recognised they deserved the same kindness and compassion and support as their daughter.

Eventually the time came, when, with the introduction of a safer, more sophisticated tracheostomy device, she was able to spend increasing amounts of time at home. On the initial visits, I heard how Rebecca was fascinated by the flames of the coal fire that heated the living room there. Such ordinary things were like magic after her long hospital confinement. The final step in her rehabilitation was a trip to a national centre, where delicate surgery successfully recreated a normal airway.

I still remember her fondly. Hopefully, her irrepressible personality and the love she received overcame any of the potential negative effects of her early experiences. I realise that, sadly, on those days when she was so frustrated, the only way she could get control of her life was to put it in danger. Paediatrics, I was learning, was a different challenge to adult medicine.

Choices

As I neared the end of the undergraduate course, I debated which direction my career should now take. Some six years before, at my admission interview, the Dean of the medical school asked me why I had chosen to study medicine. Although I knew this question was likely to come up, no-one had given me any advice as to how I might answer. I didn't come from a medical family, so if my application was successful, I would be the first in mine to study medicine. I had not, like some candidates, dreamed of being a doctor since childhood, or decided on the career because a relative had been seriously ill or died. I was not entranced by the status or salary.

I opted to tell the truth, that I wanted to learn how to treat sick people and help them recover. I wished to do something useful and beneficial for those around me. I wanted to be a healer and a scientist. I wanted to be able to look back on my life one day and say, "That was worthwhile." I worried that these ideas would sound pretentious and naively altruistic, so I was unsure how to strike a balance in describing my hopes and dreams.

I'm not certain what exactly I replied when the moment arrived, but I do remember discussing the sorts of books I read in response to a question about my general interests. I avoided mentioning thrillers and James Bond spy novels, concentrating, with encouragement, on those that had influenced my career decision. These were biographies of people like Marie Curie, Sigmund Freud, and Albert Schweitzer. We possibly talked about *The Citadel* by AJ Cronin, a novel about a young doctor in a poor Welsh mining community, and *Arrowsmith* by Sinclair Lewis, a novel about the successes and failures of a brilliant medical researcher, thwarted by society. The Dean, I realised later, had his own cunning methods of assessing applicants and getting the measure of the person in front of him; in my case, by exploring my literary interests. Somehow, I passed his test.

Meeting patients like Rebecca rekindled my long-held dreams and ambitions, which had almost become subjugated by long hours of study, especially in those early years.

Finals and the future

The process for securing a clinical post after qualification in 1970 was rather vague. It was open to everyone to apply for House jobs in any of the hospitals connected to the medical school. The selection process was allegedly fair, although not exactly transparent. Indeed, the allocation of positions seemed almost to be self-selection. It was common knowledge that, to obtain a post in one of the two major teaching hospitals, applicants probably needed to have been placed in the top quartile in the Final Examinations. It also helped if an applicant was known to the consultants in the hospital to which they applied. There were two or three units and specialties in which I was interested as possible areas in which my future career might develop. I had realised that it was wise, when on student attachment in these places, to not only be enthusiastic but to be visible, useful... and to appear competent.

In the final year of study, there were periods of time set aside in the curriculum that could be used to gain further experience in a particular field. This was to enable students who were weak in some areas to improve their knowledge and skills. The more cunning of us contrived to spend these elective attachments in units and hospitals which we favoured for house physician or surgeon posts.

As the final examinations approached, there were prize examinations in major subjects. There was only one winner in each, and in some the prize was a gold medal, depending on the generosity of the associated endowment. These medal examinations were optional and more challenging than those set by the University to assess core knowledge and diagnostic ability, and so were only taken by more confident or deluded students. Some entered without any expectation of success but as a test run for the professional exam, others did so to flag up their interest in a subject. There was considerable kudos for winners, who were guaranteed a job in the related area. The gold medal competitions identified high fliers, while the final degree examination measured competence, clinical skill, and an ability to practice safely.

I employed a strategy to target areas where the experience gained would help me decide on my eventual career direction. As I had hoped, I acquitted myself reasonably well in the general medicine, surgery and paediatric medal examinations. My chances of actually winning the paediatric gold medal floundered when I was unable to identify a peculiar rash and symptom complex in a rather irritable child. I was to learn that the unfortunate infant suffered from Pink Disease, a condition caused by Mercury poisoning, which I had never seen before, nor indeed since. The source of the Mercury was apparently in a proprietary teething powder sold exclusively by a rural pharmacist.

In the General Medicine medal examination, a rather clumsy examination technique was my downfall. I was asked to comment on some raised red oval swellings on a gentleman's shins. Intrigued, I looked carefully at his legs, then gently, or so I thought, I touched one of the lumps. The patient nearly jumped from the bed with a cry of pain. Belatedly, the penny dropped, I made the diagnosis and tried to salvage the situation. "Ah!" I said," I believe these are examples of Erythema Nodosum, possibly due to a streptococcal infection or perhaps associated with tuberculosis."

Noticing the examiner's and patient's shared pained expression I added belatedly, "the skin nodules are often exquisitely tender to the touch." He nodded and we moved on to another patient.

Croix de guerre

I entered the Psychiatry medal examination because I felt my experience in that field was less than adequate. The short taught course consisted mainly of lectures by a rather flamboyant, long-haired professor who seemed to have little personal connection with the few patients we were permitted to meet with him. Indeed, the only one I remember was an elderly gentleman from whom I was asked to elicit a history. In the course of discussing the reason for his hospital admission, he told me in rather grandiose and cultured tones that it was because he had been badly wounded and lost a leg in the second world war and coincidentally had been decorated for bravery. I enquired which award he had received. He fixed me with his eye, and replied, "The

42

Croix de Guerre, the Victoria Cross and the Iron Cross with Gold Leaf Cluster."

Surprised by his answer, which was clearly delusional, I foolishly enquired, "Which army were you fighting for?"

"Isn't it obvious?" he said, as he pulled up his trouser leg revealing, to my consternation, that he did actually have an artificial leg. "The Irish Army of course."

On the night before that examination, my revision consisted of a rapid read through a flimsy volume entitled *Lecture Notes in Psychiatry*. After the written paper, only the top 10 candidates went forward to the clinical section. To my surprise, I was selected and brought to meet a patient who had been admitted after a suicide attempt. I spent a long hour in discussion with a rather withdrawn and timid young man. It was clear to me that he was quite depressed. Later my examiners asked me if I had been able to elicit any causative or precipitating factors for his mental state in my discussions. I expanded on various avenues I had explored with him and concluded that I believed his depression was endogenous, related to his low self-esteem and introspective personality. The cool professor enquired if the young man was sexually experienced. I was rather taken aback by this question, on a topic which I had omitted to evaluate. Making the mistake of attempting to bluff, I suggested there was nothing remarkable in this area, suggesting I did not believe he currently had a girlfriend possibly due to his lack of self-confidence.

"Is it possible," said my interrogator, "that his homosexuality while living at home in a devout Christian family might have caused him some emotional distress?"

With a sinking feeling, I conceded this might be possible. I was thanked for taking part in the examination as he rose and ushered me out. I heard nothing further. I reflected that Freud would have not made the same mistake and consoled myself that, in any case, I had not been considering a career in psychiatry

The final degree examinations were considerably more straightforward. The key test was to spend an hour with a patient and diagnose their complaint. I was appreciative of patients who were keen to be helpful and almost colluded in guiding me towards the correct diagnosis, one even tipping me off that I had got it right, as the examiners approached her bed to hear my conclusion. This was a lady awaiting surgery for what I had concluded was bowel cancer, based on her symptoms and family history. It was my practice, after collecting all the relevant facts and completing the examination of a patient, to ask if there were any questions they might like to ask. She looked at me with a conspiring smile and asked, "Doctor, what exactly is a polyp?"

She had been warned not to reveal her diagnosis directly but was aware familial bowel polyps could become cancerous and was confirming my unspoken conclusion, which I then presented with confidence.

A friend had a less helpful patient who had been admitted with difficulty breathing. His answers were generally ambiguous or unhelpful. Eventually he asked the man, "Are you being treated for a heart or a chest problem?"

He replied, "Well, that's for me to know and you to find out. You're the one trying to become a doctor."

Eventually he worked out which system was causing the symptoms and passed.

Results

On a fateful afternoon in early June, the seventy men and twenty-five women who had spent six years studying together, gathered at five o'clock in front of the black-and-white entrance hall of the university's grand Lanyon Building. The Dean of the faculty, wearing his academic robes, appeared on the steps. All was silent, except for the rustle of the wind in the trees and a murmur of passing traffic in the distance.

The Dean began to read aloud, without amplification, announcing the results in alphabetical order. Residing, as I did, in the last third of the alphabet, the delay until he reached my name was torture. For each individual, the Dean listed the subjects in which the person had passed and whether they had passed with distinction. It was required to pass in each of medicine, surgery, and obstetrics. He did not indicate directly if a subject had been failed - instead omitting the subject altogether. So, for him to say only, "pass in medicine, pass in surgery," before moving on, meant the person had failed the obstetric component, which they would have to retake in the autumn. Such unfortunate news, when it arrived, caused a collective intake of breath but no-one, even then, dared to speak. Omitting a name altogether indicated failure in all subjects. The Dean only paused in his delivery after announcing someone had passed with honours, which required a distinction mark in all three subjects. This short delay was to allow a brief cheer and applause. He knew how to work his audience, and the tension held. It was only when he finished speaking that we realised that a few of our number had failed, and the fact that, personally, I had passed, fully sank in.

Then it was off to the pub.

A short time later, I phoned home from a call box to report the good news. Even later I drove back to the house to be congratulated by my family. As my mother kissed and hugged me, she drew back.

"Have you been drinking?" she asked, shocked. My parents were strictly teetotal and liked to believe their children followed their example. Assuring her it was just a celebratory drink, I headed back to join my friends again. Much later, some of us were ejected from the pub for anti-social behaviour - in my case, for lying on my back on a table, one of several people competing in an upside down, imaginary cycling race while a noisy crowd decided which participant's legs were moving fastest.

Even later, I went to see my girlfriend, who was house-sitting for her aunt while she was abroad on holiday. Eventually, I was admitted - if only because my persistent knocking and ringing of the doorbell was in danger of waking the neighbourhood. Ignoring all protests, I staggered upstairs.

I awoke the following afternoon to find I was lying on a bed, still fully clothed, including jacket, trousers, socks and shoes. I received no sympathy for my self-inflicted state and learned that once I had reached the horizontal position I had lapsed into unconsciousness. My girlfriend's virtue was intact, but I felt as if I had suffered a craniotomy.

The following Monday, I set about securing my first choice hospital posts.

Like most of the general population, many medical students regarded surgeons as being at the top of the professional pyramid - a concept promoted by film and television portrayals of handsome macho characters and documentaries with titles such as 'Your Life in Their Hands'. I was equally impressed by the real life professors of medicine I had encountered, one of whom had encouraged me to undertake a short research project in his laboratory. Ultimately, I was persuaded by the gentle, empathetic personalities that seemed characteristic of paediatricians - and by the vulnerability of their patients - to consider exploring children's medicine as an option.

So, smartly dressed, I approached the professor of paediatrics and the senior surgeon, whom I had admired since our encounter with the unfortunate alcoholic. He had combined kindness rather than arrogance with his operative skill. I politely explained to them that I was applying to their hospital for a house post and would be honoured to be allocated to their unit, should I be successful. They both responded with the standard form of words explaining that, while they could guarantee nothing until the appointment committee met, they hoped they would see me in the autumn. I felt my reception had been positive. There was a saying in those days that, "job canvassing disqualifies and not canvassing definitely disqualifies".

Having done my best to at least declare my interests, and after submitting the official application document, I departed with five newly-qualified friends for a well earned holiday, taking a rented motor cruiser, sometimes precariously, down the rivers and loughs of Ireland. Our last summer free of responsibility.

Looking back

Reflecting on my student years, lights up a kaleidoscope of vivid memories, some of which I have related.

There was the shock of my first encounter with death and dying.

Recollections of particular patients, their diagnoses, personalities, and differing responses to becoming ill.

My initial experiences of how different nurses and doctors coped with human tragedy, with distraught families, their tears and distress, and of wondering how I would manage when called upon to do the same.

Memories of agonising for patients faced with the knowledge their life was under threat, sympathising with their initial fear, resentment, resignation - and sometimes being privileged to watch as they found a courage they never knew they possessed.

I was humbled by how many, when seriously ill, worried more for their families than for themselves. I came to respect people coping with the worst days of their lives, which strengthened a desire to help them as best I could.

There was the drama of cardiac resuscitation and emergency surgery.

The keenly felt injustice of illness in children.

These things, and of course the exhilaration of seeing lives saved, pain relieved, and the elation of being part of a skilled treatment team, confirmed for me that I had chosen the right career.

The gift of seeing many people recover to full health and appreciating the relief this brought - not just to them, but to those close to them.

The demands of learning and understanding routine treatment for common ailments and taking pleasure in observing the expected response.

Days working towards academic success against a niggling fear of failure, relieved by glorious nights of partying, and years of camaraderie and friendship.

Days spent seeking out those with every variety of symptoms or signs of disease: Heart murmurs and heart failure, tremors and patterns of paralysis, enlarged livers, abdominal masses, kidney stones and gallstones, arthritic joints, varicose veins, wheezing chests and shortness of breath. Each of us hoping we could recognise any disease presented to us in the final examinations.

Into our heads, we crammed knowledge of anatomy, physiology, pharmacology, therapeutics, microbiology, infectious diseases, psychiatry, neurology, cardiology, obstetrics, gynaecology and more. Everything that would entitle us, after six years of study, to call ourselves doctors.

The new house doctor I became was a different person, in many ways, from the individual who left school at 18. Exposure to alternative outlooks on life, scientific methodology and thinking; to teachers, fellow students and,

47

most of all, to patients from diverse social, religious, political and academic backgrounds created a more impartial and self-critical person.

3. House doctor

Paediatrics

My first post as a doctor was a three-month spell in the paediatric academic unit. My little friend Rebecca was still there, awaiting the surgery which would soon change her life and allow her to go home at last. Most of the patients had been admitted with common acute conditions - chest infections, severe asthma, seizures due to epilepsy or a neurological disorder. Others had bowel disorders, such as coeliac disease caused by wheat gluten allergy. A significant proportion, though, had more serious problems. Several had cystic fibrosis, diabetes, and a variety of haematological disorders, including acute leukaemia. On my first day, the professor made several things clear to the new junior staff.

Firstly, we must never be too embarrassed to ask for help.

Next, with every decision we made, we must ensure that the children in our care stayed safe. He pointed out that his unit had over 30 beds and cots so, if we were uncertain if a patient's condition warranted admission, we could err on the safe side and bring them in for observation. He, or another consultant, would be happy to review each admission later. This sort of safety net is no longer available in many areas of the health service, with the insidious reduction in bed numbers.

Ivo, as we referred to him when he was not around, was an approachable, pragmatic and compassionate man. He never seemed to get outwardly upset. He proved to be a supportive mentor and teacher.

I became alert to the possibility that an unexplained fever in a small child might turn out to be the only early sign of meningitis. Effective vaccines had yet to make a significant preventative impact on the incidence of this condition. So another of Ivo's safety rules was that any child under the age of one year who had a seizure precipitated by a high temperature would have to have a lumbar puncture to exclude the possibility of this dangerous infection. I soon became adept at performing the procedure.

As a pre-registration house physician, most of my work was supervised, at least initially, by supportive senior colleagues. There was a lot to learn, but there was also a great team spirit - and older trainees were generally ready with help and advice.

I was protected from making life and death decisions, which I understood some of my first year colleagues faced elsewhere. In paediatrics, there were always two doctors with more experience than me around, day and night. There was little talk of stress, or anxiety amongst us - and nights with little sleep were accepted as part of the job.

I spent a lot of time taking children's medical histories, recording medical admission details and ward round decisions. Gradually, I learnt how to put small children, and even parents, at ease as we talked. An important, but time consuming, daily job was drawing blood samples. Many children had a fear of needles, so I was thankful for effective anaesthetic ointment and numbing alcohol skin sprays. The children responded best to kindness, sympathy and humour. I discovered many, often the sickest, refused to complain, even when questioned. The children never ceased to surprise me with their innate sense of fun and mischief. Turning tests, such as radiological examinations, into a game became a challenge. Of necessity, avoiding incomprehensible medical jargon became a habit. An anatomy lecturer had once informed us that, by the time we graduated, we would have doubled our vocabulary. In paediatrics, we needed to use the simplest words. Fancy anatomical terminology had no place here. I tried to talk simply and listen to my small charges. The younger ones found the use of terms like, bottom, bum, poo, or wee, hilarious, but they knew what we meant. In contrast, an older boy who had his appendix removed in an adult ward in another hospital, was asked by the nurses on several succeeding mornings if his bowels had moved. Worried, he checked his testicles each time, since they were just below his operation wound, and answered, "No". Eventually, when in danger of receiving large doses of laxatives, someone explained this strange question was not in fact an inquiry about his balls, but was inquiring whether he had passed a motion. Simple terms worked best.

The tightrope walkers

One of my fairly regular tasks was the intravenous administration of Cryoprecipitate to boys with haemophilia. This was a blood plasma fraction containing a concentration of the clotting factor which patients born with this condition lack. This was usually required because some minor trauma had caused bleeding. What might cause an insignificant bruise in other children could result in considerable blood loss into the tissues of affected boys. It was most important to speedily arrest bleeding in the muscles and joints to avoid permanent damage and limitation of mobility.

There were a couple of brothers with this condition whom I got to know. They were, I think, farmer's sons and frequently seemed to be up to some escapade which resulted in a ward visit.

One weekend they were taken to see a travelling circus and, on returning home, decided to emulate the tightrope walkers who had impressed them. They reckoned the trick couldn't be very difficult and fixed a sturdy rope between two barns. All seemed to be going well as the older boy edged out along the rope until his brother, watching his success, decided to follow. The metre-long fall onto the farmyard below was inevitable. Several days of hospital treatment were necessary because of traumatic bleeding into the knee and wrist joints. They quickly become bored. With a dairy farm to manage and other children at home, their parents found it difficult to be constantly present to keep them occupied or amused. On their third or fourth evening with us, the hospital received a phone call from the barman in the Beehive Pub, which was just across the busy road, almost opposite the hospital.

"I've two young lads here asking to use the phone to call a taxi to take them home. For a start they only have one pound eighty pence between them - and one of the customers has recognised them from the hospital. I've given them a bottle of Coke and a bag of crisps each and told them I would see what I could do. They think I'm on the phone to a taxi company. I expect you will want to send someone to collect them."

After a quick discussion, the night sister and a porter were dispatched. The boys got a great cheer from the lads in the bar as they left. The parents were shocked at first, then relieved when reassured that the boys had come to no harm. They may have been a little impressed and amused by their daring but, if they were, they didn't give it away to the boys, with whom they were extremely cross. Fortunately, litigation was not even considered. Times would change.

"Boys will be boys, but this mustn't ever happen again," said their father apologetically, when they eventually left us. Today, the doors to children's wards are kept locked.

Cryoprecipitate, which was prepared from locally-donated blood, was later replaced by a smaller volume of injectable Clotting Factor VIII Concentrate, often sourced from North America. Tragically, viral contamination of this product was responsible for large numbers of recipients becoming infected with the Hepatitis and HIV viruses, with devastating results. The Cryoprecipitate was, in contrast, safe and caused no such infections.

Casualty, rubber bullets, and internment

In 1971, in the strongly republican area outside the hospital, the Troubles raged - but the children's ward was almost a place of sanctuary from the violence. In the children's casualty department, we not only treated accident and emergency cases but also functioned as an out-of-hours medical service. Not many family doctors were keen to do house calls after dark, as had been past practice, when rioting and car hijacking were relatively frequent occurrences.

The variety of patients I saw made the work there fascinating. Ill babies were alarming as they seemed so frail. During one of my first experiences of managing alone, a small child was carried in, still in a violent seizure. I remembered immediately my shock on observing a similar event as a student, and the effective intravenous injection employed. This time, the same drug failed to stop the fit. I decided I should try giving a drug called paraldehyde, which was administered rectally. It is a toxic medicine which must be drawn up in a glass syringe as it could damage the rubber plunger of standard plastic syringes. The fit subsided, leaving the aroma of paraldehyde in the air and on the child's breath. This form of a treatment is no longer employed. Buccal Midazolam, a drug related to Valium that can be rapidly absorbed from the lining of the mouth is highly effective, and has become the preferred treatment.

Over the following weeks, I emulated the performance of the skilled and experienced senior nurses, learning how to appear calm and, eventually, actually acting as calmly as they generally did in a fraught situation.

At other times we got some amusement from inappropriately worried mothers. Of course, we hid this to avoid offence. One woman was in a terrible state when she arrived with her thee-year-old son, whom she had discovered eating her packet of contraceptive pills.

"What will they do to his dicky bird?" she asked, close to tears. "Will it turn him into a wee girl?"

Checking the blister pack revealed that he had only eaten two oestrogen tablets, so we were able to reassure her that at worst they might make him nauseous for a short time, but he would come to no long-term harm.

It was relatively common for children to arrive having consumed a variety of medications. Quite often, these were colourful pills counted and set out in a bedroom by visiting grandparents, for consumption at bedtime. Heart or blood pressure drugs, and even iron tablets, are potentially very dangerous to small children.

A standard first line treatment given to children who had ingested these potential poisons, was a dose of Syrup of Ipecacuanha. This was an effective plant based emetic, causing vomiting shortly after being administered. It was taught that this undoubtedly limited the absorption of the poison. I was impressed by its dramatic effect. There were limitations to its use, however. For example, it was not given if the ingested material was caustic or oily. It seemed to be a simple and palatable prescription until, disappointingly, rigorous scientific studies demonstrated that, in fact, it did not consistently remove poisons from the stomach or reliably prevent their absorption. It was replaced, in some instances, by equally unpleasant stomach washouts, administered via a tube passed through the nose into the stomach. Activated charcoal might be left behind to bind to the chemical and, where possible, specific antidotes became a chosen treatment.

The advent of child-proof packaging in the late 1970s saw a dramatic drop in these sorts of admissions. Before the advent of "child-proof" locking bottle tops for dangerous liquids, however, I saw the devastating, life-threatening effect on a boy of drinking a mouthful of a caustic cleaning fluid which had been stored in an old corked bottle. He only survived after major reconstructive surgery to replace his ruined oesophagus with a transposed section of bowel.

Some problems were more easily resolved. A panicked mum brought in a tiny child who she swore had a moth bite on his nose. She had seen the creature sitting on his face when she checked him in his cot. She was worried it might have been poisonous. The dark dot on his nose, pointed out as evidence, was easily wiped off. She left greatly relieved, having had it confirmed that our local moths could not bite.

A struggling boy was carried in with the help of two ambulance men. He had prised open the join on the side of some bathroom weighing scales in order to look inside and see how they worked. Unable to keep holding the top and bottom sections apart, he wedged them open by inserting his foot in between, where it became trapped. Fortunately, a hospital maintenance engineer was able to cut into the metal and open the gap further with some tools. The released foot, although painful, had only superficial abrasions through his sock.

The casualty sister kept a display of strange items which had been removed from inquisitive children and those bathroom scales held pride of place, alongside a saucepan which a boy had wedged on his head. Such boys took some pride in their short-lived notoriety.

On another occasion, a toddler was brought along having managed to pick the diamond out of his mother's engagement ring and push it up his nose before anyone could stop him. Using a nasal speculum to gently widen his nostril, I located the precious stone and attempted to remove it using long, slim forceps. At the crucial moment I gripped it, he wriggled in his mum's arms, despite the assistance of a nurse who was holding him steady. The gem shot from the tip of the forceps further up his nose and out of sight. The Nose and Throat Specialist later retrieved it, with the little lad asleep under anaesthesia. I decided not to confess that I'd made matters worse. The diamond was not retained for the display cabinet.

One evening, I was confronted by a couple of grubby boys who were maybe nine or ten years old.

"Doctor, would you like to buy a rubber bullet?" one of them asked. I was astounded as he held the black object out. It was about the size of the small one-third pint bottles of milk given out in schools until Mrs. Thatcher stopped this largesse. They were hard, ugly objects about 15 cm long and 4 cm in diameter. After some bartering, I parted with 50 pence. I asked where they had found the ammunition.

"If you are quick you can pick up one or two lying around after a riot," one volunteered with a grin, while pocketing the money.

"Look boys, for God's sake, get home out of the way if there is any trouble in the streets. I don't want to see you in here again having been hit by one of these."

"Wise up, Doc, do you think we're daft?"

I wondered how many bullets these young entrepreneurs had collected and sold.

My accommodation was in the East Wing of the hospital complex and looked out over the Lower Falls and Grosvenor Roads. On the evening of the 9th August 1971, I stood on the roof of the building. From early morning, the streets opposite the hospital had been virtually sealed off by troops and police. It was the end of our first week as newly qualified doctors. We felt cut off from the town, inside the hospital - but the early morning the sound of dustbin lids being hammered on the ground alerted us, and those living in the houses opposite, that the Royal Ulster Constabulary, supported by the British Army, was moving into the area in force. As dusk fell, a few of us were curious to see what exactly was happening, but not foolish enough to venture out into the streets.

We knew the building well, having lived there for many months as senior medical students in training. We located the maintenance stairwell to the roof and discreetly slipped out into the shelter of a parapet or chimney stack to have a look. The area below was cordoned off by roadblocks. Any car approaching the road into the hospital was being stopped and searched, to deter any through traffic, and to block anyone attempting to escape the area through the hospital's rear exit. The intermittent banging of metal bin lids and the presence of troops and army vehicles on the ground had created an air of menace. Residents had blocked some side streets with improvised barricades and hijacked cars. In the distance, dark smoke rose into the dusk, possibly from a burning bus. The sight of cars, taxis and even private ambulances fleeing the area confirmed that this was not a simple raid targeted on a single individual. As we peered out across Dunville Park, which is opposite the hospital, towards Leeson Street, we reckoned from previous experience that the casualty department would have a busy night.

We were only watching for a few minutes when a bright light swept along the roof. As we ducked back inside, an English voice came over a loud hailer.

"Retire immediately from the rooftop of the hospital or your lives may be in danger. I repeat, you must leave the rooftop immediately."

Shocked, we stampeded back down the stairs, slamming the access door behind us as the voice repeated in the distance, "You must leave the rooftop at once!"

Somebody said, "Thank God we kept our white coats on."

This was the beginning of the infamous internment strategy, which led to a total of 342 men being arrested and imprisoned without trial, in a misguided effort by the authorities to halt the downward spiral of violence in the city.

Inside the hospital, the staff continued to work and look after our patients as usual, while outside, especially after dark, the atmosphere was often tense. Despite the civil unrest, it was rare for anyone not to turn in for work as usual, no matter what their role in the hospital, or where they lived in the city. Staff at every level took a pride in carrying on, regardless of barricades and bombs.

A peculiar smell

As I arrived in the ward one morning towards the end of my stint in paediatrics I detected a pleasant odour in the air. Although it seemed vaguely familiar, I could not place what it was.

"What is that peculiar smell in the corridor?" I asked the ward sister.

"Oh, we had a child admitted with Croup last night. We're steaming him with Friar's Balsam. It's an old traditional remedy."

She handed me a small bottle. The label described the contents as a tincture of aromatic benzoic compounds.

"The Balsam is added to the water in the special kettle which is heated to boiling point. Inhaling the vapour is supposed to be great for opening up the bronchial tubes. Mind you, if you're in the room for very long, the smell tends to cling to your clothes all day."

I realised why I liked the smell, which most of the staff were turning their noses up at. A memory flooded back from my toddler years, when I had been briefly in hospital. I had heard the story from my mother on many occasions. I had developed the crowing inspiratory croak of croup, caused by a viral inflammation swelling and narrowing the upper airway. The strange stridor scared my parents so much, they feared I would stop breathing. A vague recollection awakened of sitting on a bed, surrounded by greenish curtains, a large kettle with a long spout nearby, emitting steam suffused with this peculiar smell. I reflected that the Friar's Balsam must have given me some relief and created a positive association with this unique odour.

I stepped into the side ward to talk to the toddler and his mother. After listening to his chest, I concluded his breathing difficulty was less laboured than had been recorded when he was admitted. I told them the story of my own experience of croup to reassure them he should be well very soon. Indeed, within a couple of days he was discharged, his breathing back to normal. Eventually, the use of Friars Balsam was superseded by a truly effective treatment in the form of a single anti-inflammatory dose of the steroid dexamethasone. This drug is now widely known as a key part of the treatment of critical respiratory inflammation caused by the COVID-19 virus.

My three-month rotation through paediatrics was drawing to a close. I had become relatively expert at taking blood samples and inserting intravenous cannulas into small veins. Skills which would subsequently come in useful when I returned to the adult wards. I was occasionally called upon by other junior colleagues having difficulty gaining venous access, who knew of my experience.

Caring for children who suffered from life limiting conditions in that first ward made a deep impression. I had made the transition from student to doctor, and from observer to full participant in the treatment and lives of patients. I had come to realise that doctors are part of a team composed of other professional colleagues, parents and families.

I now had first-hand experience of children born in the decade prior to 1970 with the inherited disease cystic fibrosis, at a time when less than 25 percent were likely to survive to adulthood. In time, I got to know a few who had fought through that chronic illness to become teenagers. They had the same hopes and dreams as their friends - but unspoken between us was the knowledge they were unlikely to achieve many of these. I admired their spirit, and that of their parents, but I did not have the experience or a close enough relationship to broach such a sensitive subject with them. The outlook for cystic fibrosis patients is dramatically different today.

Similarly, over half of the children I met in those first months who had developed acute leukaemia, would die, most only surviving a few years. Thankfully, with modern chemotherapy and other treatments, this is no longer the case.

At the same time, I was inspired by the ability of most children to bounce back from acute illness and also by the love of parents I saw each day. It was a delight to discover that toddlers will smile when you smile, laugh when you laugh - and if you can win that smile and laugh, they may even forgive you for the upset of the last blood test. I had learnt to try to listen to children and address their worries, not just those of their parents. I loved those three months and so I was already considering that this might be where my future lay, but I was yet to experience adult medicine and surgery, at first hand.

Neurology

"You will need to complete a death certificate," said my new ward Sister, unlocking a drawer in her desk. She withdrew a large, official beige book of certificates and placed it in front of me. I protested that I barely knew the patient and suggested the paperwork should be completed by someone more senior.

She sat down, straightening her crisp white apron, and smoothing the crinkles in her red dress. I looked at the attractive dark haired nurse who was rumoured to be doing a steady romantic line with a senior registrar in the hospital.

"The houseman always issues the death certificates, once they have seen the body," she said sympathetically.

"I'm sorry, it's just that I've never filled one out before and I need to be careful and think about the correct terms to use."

Her face showed surprise at this.

"You have been in post for over three months and have never needed to fill out a death certificate?"

I confirmed this, and for the first time it registered with me that in the children's ward I had not had to cope directly with a single death. The loss of a child is devastating for everyone involved, including nurses and doctors. Had my older colleagues possibly protected me from this experience? I didn't think so, it was just that a senior doctor, usually a consultant, dealt with grieving parents. Adult medicine was clearly going to be different. Here, the majority of patients were elderly and in the neurology ward, where I had been working for only a week, several patients had chronic, progressive or degenerative conditions. All had diseases of the brain, spinal cord or peripheral nervous system.

When I first encountered Mr Currie and his family, he was already extremely weak, his breathing shallow and laboured. He had developed pneumonia, complicating his advanced motor neurone disease. There was no cure for this condition, which leads to progressive loss of muscle function. He even had difficulty swallowing his saliva and had refused to be fed through a nasogastric tube. He made it clear he did not wish his chest infection to be treated with antibiotics. His wife and family had held vigil with him, as the nurses made him as comfortable as possible, while he gradually lapsed into unconsciousness and slipped away.

I completed the certificate and checked with a friend who held the post before me that I had used the legally correct terminology. Sister then accompanied me to sit down with the family to listen to them talk about the husband and father they had lost. I learned from her a little of how to deal kindly and professionally with mourning relatives, a difficult role for which most new doctors felt ill-prepared. How best to communicate bad or sad news was not something we had learned as students. When the family were ready to leave, I shook hands with each one and offered my sympathy. After they had gone, I reflected that this man was no older than my own father. Today medical schools offer training modules on breaking bad news. It remains a difficult task.

A ruined Christmas dinner

I was now working in a non-acute ward, with most patients booked in for assessment and diagnosis. The majority of my duties were therefore routine, making notes of consultants' comments and orders, arranging tests and collating results. However, my experience of performing lumbar punctures (LPs) on children, to exclude the possibility of meningitis, proved invaluable in my new unit. Each Friday afternoon, I would routinely be sent individuals from my consultant's clinic to have this diagnostic procedure performed. This was to obtain spinal fluid samples for analysis. Although initially a rather frightening prospect for patients, once some local anaesthetic was infiltrated in the appropriate lumbar area, the process of passing a needle through a vertebral disc space into the fluid in the spinal canal was usually quick and only slightly uncomfortable.

On one occasion in early December, I was called upon to carry out this test on a schoolteacher in his mid-forties. He rested in the ward after the LP, as was obligatory, lying flat on a bed for a couple of hours, as this generally prevented the development of a headache which otherwise was a frequent, if minor, complication. My work for the day completed, I headed off to the resident doctor's dining room for dinner. Just as I arrived there, my pager began to bleep. I phoned the ward and an anxious nurse immediately answered.

"It's the gentleman who had the LP earlier. We have been carrying out the routine observations as requested, and it seems he has lost feeling in his legs."

Shocked and rather worried, I rushed back and examined him carefully, to check the nurse's finding. I asked him to close his eyes and touched his skin over his shins with the point of a needle, asking him to let me know each time he felt the tip. Despite multiple pricks with the increasing pressure, he gave no response. I then tested his knee and ankle reflexes with a patella hammer and found that the responses were undoubtedly weak. I explained that this was unusual and told him I was going to contact his consultant for advice. In the meantime, I advised that he should just continue to rest.

Fortunately, the consultant neurologist had not left the hospital and came to see him immediately. On confirming our conclusions, he also checked that the LP needle had been inserted into the patient's back at the correct level - that is, below the lower end of the spinal cord, which does not extend to the bottom of the bony spine. He decided that we should perform a repeat LP, but this time introduce some Myodil, a radiopaque contrast fluid, into the spinal canal. This would outline the internal structure that is normally obscured by the vertebral bone structure on a simple X-ray. He summoned a neuroradiologist from home to carry out the study, known as a myelogram. This quickly established that there was a previously unsuspected spinal tumour. He concluded that the withdrawal of spinal fluid by the first LP had caused the tumour, previously sited higher in the canal, to shift downwards and impinge on the cord.

We now had an emergency situation. Immediate surgery was essential to decompress the spinal canal, relieving pressure on the delicate spinal cord and preventing permanent damage.

My consultant went back to explain the situation to our patient.

I telephoned the specialist neurosurgeon, who was on call, at home. He was about to leave for a Christmas dinner. An anaesthetist and operating theatre team then had to be alerted. The surgeon arrived shortly in a dinner jacket and bow tie, reviewed the X-ray images, and explained to the shocked patient the nature and necessity of an operation.

As we walked away, the surgeon demanded of me, "Who in God's name carried out a lumbar puncture on a Friday afternoon?"

I confessed that it was me, and tried to explain it was on the instruction of my boss. He demanded to know where he was - fortunately, just as he entered the office. I was able to slip away.

Happily, not only was the pressure relieved, but subsequently the tumour was successfully removed. The patient did not become paralysed and gradually made a full recovery. He was well enough to be discharged in time for Christmas. I was embarrassed when, on leaving, he thanked me and offered me a present. Later, I opened it to find a large packet of 200 Sterling cigarettes. I was a non-smoker.

An unfortunate omission

It is essential that those involved in performing lumbar puncture procedures understand it is imperative that no bacteria must enter the spinal canal with the needle. One afternoon, we received a request from the School of Nursing asking if final year students might come and observe the correct aseptic technique. The tutors had noted that the topic had not come up for some years in the Royal College of Nursing Examination and predicted it might do so this time. Consent to have the student nurses present was obtained from a patient who was due to have a myelogram.This was the identical procedure to that which had identified `'s tumour. Our ward Sister volunteered to act as my assistant and talk the students through the process of setting up the instruments and providing the antiseptic solutions required by the doctor. She emphasised the nurse's role in ensuring there was meticulous attention to sterility throughout.

Sister did an excellent teaching job to which I listened intently as she described everything step by step. With the LP performed, the students left, and the obliging patient was taken off to the Neuroradiology suite. Sister and I sat down for a cup of tea but were interrupted by a phone call. I watched expressions of surprise and concern cross her face, as she spoke inaudibly into the handset. She replaced it, held up an open hand towards me, and disappeared out the door. She returned within a minute holding a vial of Myodil contrast fluid.

"The radiologist on the phone said he couldn't locate any Myodil in the spinal canal. We were so busy teaching those blessed students that, after collecting the spinal fluid sample, we both neglected to then inject dye through the needle. He has told the patient he needs to have more contrast injected in order to obtain better pictures."

I sat horrified by our omission - and possibly even swore.

Our tea abandoned, Sister rapidly set up for another LP. We apologised profusely to the patient as we repeated the procedure, this time with no students present.. Our patient made no complaint and we thanked him for being so gracious. He was taken once more on a trolley to have new images taken. As he was wheeled out, he remarked that he was pleased to have been able to do something in return for the wonderful nursing care he had experienced over previous months. We were not only embarrassed but humbled. For the rest of my tenure, Sister and I had a special, mutually supportive working relationship.

Gin and tonic

Throughout my three months as the neurology house doctor, there was a long-term patient in the unit who had suffered a catastrophic brain haemorrhage or injury, some years previously. She seemed to have no awareness of her surroundings, even when apparently awake. I was given to understand that the severity of Dorothy's disability was down to her damaged brain. Occasionally, I wondered if some of her difficulties were because she had become progressively withdrawn and dispirited. Certainly, she was unable to speak, communicate or walk. She made no attempt to read or move and required constant nursing care. Her condition had, in fact, been thoroughly evaluated and classified as a chronic vegetative state. I understood that, in the past, she had had a successful professional career. I never encountered any visitors but once spoke with a more senior colleague who had done so in the past.

"Apparently in her younger days, she enjoyed a gin and tonic," he said ruefully

I developed a habit of sitting down beside her bed for a few minutes when I carried out my night round, if she seemed to be awake. I would talk to her quietly about any topic which came into my head. These conversations were of course one-sided.

One evening, I was discussing a hospital Christmas drinks reception I had attended. Suddenly I heard myself saying, "I gather you are partial to a gin and tonic yourself."

I thought I saw a slight flicker of movement around her lips. Then it was gone. I sat looking intently at Dorothy, but although her eyes faced forward, I could not convince myself there was any significant contact with mine.

"It's nearly Christmas," I said. "I'll have to see what I can do."

I went to the doctor's bar in our living quarters, obtained an extremely small measure of gin and a bottle of tonic water. On returning to the ward, I mixed a very weak gin and tonic in a spouted drinking cup. My friend was still awake. I held the spout to her lips as I had watched the nurses do, and she gradually swallowed some of the cocktail. Officially, no one ever knew what I was up to, but the night staff may have wondered why I sometimes helped Dorothy to a drink late at night. Some may have recognised the very faint smell but said nothing. On the final day of my stint in that unit, as I showed my replacement around, we stopped briefly at her bed.

After describing her difficulties, I gave her a wink.

"By the way, Dorothy likes a weak Gin and Tonic as a nightcap now and again."

I didn't expand.

Cardio-thoracic surgery

On the night of 4 December, 1971, a bomb exploded in McGurk's bar in a Catholic area of Belfast, killing 12 people and injuring a similar number, some of them seriously. This escalation in violence was to set the tone for the next year, the worst in the Northern Irish Troubles. Almost 500 people were killed. That February, I moved to the post of house officer in surgery. On my previous stints, in paediatrics and neurology, I had not been directly involved in dealing with casualties or fatalities from the civil unrest, but I was now to come face to face with the brutality of those days.

Kicked by a horse

My first post was in a cardio-thoracic ward, where the day-to-day work was open heart surgery such as heart valve replacements and chest operations for conditions including lung cancer. Coronary bypass surgery had only just been developed.

Soon, I became adept at new procedures, such as placing or removing chest drains. These tubes were important for draining residual blood postoperatively from the thoracic cavity. When this loss tailed off, we knew things had healed internally and the tube was removed. On other occasions, they were placed to drain air leaking from a damaged or punctured lung. The end of the tube was anchored underwater in a sterile, sealed bottle. When there was such a leak, the air which had escaped outside the lung bubbled out through this water trap with each breath. We knew the air leak had sealed when the water bubbles ceased. Removing these chest drains as painlessly as possible was a particular challenge for the junior doctor.

I tried numerous manoeuvres to cause the minimum of pain when doing so, including shots of intravenous morphine immediately prior to the assault, and infiltrating local anaesthetic around the tissue at the exit site. Despite my best efforts, a County Down farmer described the experience to me as like being kicked by a horse. Matters were made worse by macho boasts in the male ward, where patients who had come through the extraction procedure, competed with each other in describing their ability to endure excruciating pain.

Eventually, I developed a new technique to combine with the analgesia and anaesthesia. employing a variation of distraction techniques I had learnt in paediatrics. I would advise the subject to hold onto the bed frame with both hands, thus delaying any attempt to grab me or the tube. As sympathetically as possible, I would advise that I would count to five before pulling out the tube, so that they could steel themselves. I suggested this usually alleviated the discomfort. I would then proceed to slowly count aloud but yank the tube out on the number three.

I inevitably felt a little guilty, but liked to think the shock of pain was short-lived - speaking, of course, as someone who has never had a chest tube removed or been kicked by a horse.

Cow staggers

One evening, I was paged to go quickly to the casualty department by my senior registrar, Vijay, who was shortly to take up a consultant post. A soldier was being rushed in by ambulance, having been shot through the chest by a sniper using a high velocity rifle. When the victim arrived, he was semi-conscious, his breathing was shallow and his pulse rate and blood pressure critically low. The emergency trauma team leapt into action. His flak jacket and clothes were cut off to reveal a small entrance hole on the front of his chest and a much larger ragged exit wound in his back. These were immediately cleaned and dressed as the resuscitation team worked frantically. My minor job was to take a blood sample and get it to the blood bank for the cross matching of six units. I was also instructed to contact the consultant thoracic surgeon on call, while Vijay placed a chest drain and, with the others, worked to get the patient stable enough to transfer him to the operating theatre, which was already standing by to receive him.

The senior surgeon's wife answered the phone immediately but, to my amazement, informed me that her husband was dealing with some sick cows. I later learned he was administering injections of magnesium sulphate into the jugular veins of his prize herd, to treat grass staggers. A low magnesium level in young cattle can apparently cause fits and death. When I explained the reason for my call, she assured me she knew exactly where he was, it was close by, and guaranteed he would be on his way within minutes.

I then headed for the theatre, where an anaesthetist was placing an endotracheal tube into the soldier's windpipe so that the mechanical ventilator could take over his breathing as he slipped into painless unconsciousness. A message came through from our ward to say the consultant surgeon had left home and would be with us in about 10 minutes. He sent instructions that Vijay, who was meticulously scrubbing up, should start the operation. I was to scrub up to assist him, if necessary. The operating theatre Sister and two nurses were already gowned up and setting out the contents of the sterile thoracotomy instrument pack. As Vijay and I pulled on our sterile gowns, donned hats, masks and gloves, the door swung open and another senior surgeon appeared. He had been operating next door.

"Right," he announced. "I'm here now and will take over. Vijay, you can assist me."

Vijay explained our consultant was arriving at any minute - and had instructed that he should start the procedure if everything was ready to go before he arrived.

"Fine! Fine! Let's get started then" he barked, lathering his hands and arms in soap, followed by iodine antiseptic solution.

"You," he said, looking at me. "Let your consultant know I'm here and he does not need to worry any further about this case."

Shortly, as they waited for the anaesthetist to be satisfied he had good venous access, and for the various monitors to indicate cardiovascular stability, my boss appeared beside me. I explained, as he washed his hands, about the Professor being present next door.

"Savage," he said. "Get in there and tell him I am here, and Vijay is to start the surgery as I instructed. He is more than capable, as we both know. We do not need any outside help."

I drew a deep breath and went to speak to the Professor, trying to deliver the message with due deference.

"I don't think you have explained things properly," he said to me testily.

"Vijay is indeed about to operate, and I will be assisting him." This was a tactical role reversal.

I heard the door behind me being kicked open. My boss entered, preceded by his gloved hands. I saw his eyes narrow. From behind his surgical mask, he spoke.

"Thanks for your help, but now, you can get the hell out of my Theatre!"

He was not speaking to me, but I left discreetly and waited for a few minutes in the adjacent anaesthetic room before returning to observe my two senior colleagues work with exceptional speed and skill.

Rapidly, the chest was opened, the internal bleeding arrested, and the trauma caused by the bullet to the lung and chest wall expertly repaired.

The soldier was in the intensive care unit for several days before returning to us. While he recovered, in a room off our main ward, a discreet armed guard was placed at the entrance until he was well enough to be transferred to the nearby military hospital.

The soldier never knew of the mini macho side drama that took place as his life hung in the balance, and he didn't utter a sound as I pulled the chest drains.

The clot

"Well, young man," snarled the heart surgeon at me, "you're in shit aren't you son?"

We looked each other straight in the eye. No doctor had ever spoken to me like this before. My scalp tingled, my mouth was dry. Shocked, I took a deep breath.

Since the ward sister informed me a few minutes earlier that he wanted to see me as soon as I appeared, I had been re-examining, in my mind, the events which had started at 3 o'clock that morning.

My boss was highly respected for his extraordinary operating skill, but also well known for his occasionally volatile and abrasive manner. The speed at which he was chewing gum at this moment was a measure of his level of agitation. As a result of this, I was being subjected to the sharp end of his tongue. Intimidated by his language, I concentrated on remaining outwardly calm and rational as I recalled the events of the previous night.

When the phone rang in the early hours, I was fast asleep in the hot, stuffy room I had been allocated for my year as a house doctor. Of course, I might perhaps have tried opening the sash window to admit some fresh air, but only with a superhuman effort, since it has been painted shut several times. My single bed was pressed tight against the wall, otherwise it would have been impossible to fully open the door. The other floor space was occupied by ancient furniture: A well worn desk, a wonky wardrobe, a battered armchair and a small bedside cabinet, on which resided a lamp and the phone. I felt around in the darkness and only succeeded in knocking the handset from the cradle. Switching on the light, the bilious green NHS decor was illuminated as my radio bleep went off

"Hello," I said, having located the phone. A bright friendly female voice answered.

"Did I wake you?" the nurse at the other end inquired. I failed to resist the urge for sarcasm.

"No of course not, I'm always entertaining friends and enjoying myself at this time of night."

"There's no need to be a smart Alec," she replied. "I hope it's not that poor innocent girl I see you chatting up in the Dungeon."

The Dungeon was the aptly named underground canteen in the depths of the hospital. I did not rise to the bait but asked if she had something more important to discuss.

"Yes, actually, I think Mrs. O'Leary in the side ward has a deep vein thrombosis in her left leg. Her calf muscle is painful, and her ankle looks a bit swollen. Would you mind having a look?"

I dropped the banter, agreed to be straight there, and hung up.

Releasing a weary groan, I got up, splashed some water on my face, applied some deodorant, and quickly dressed. I jogged down three flights of stairs, then walked along the eerily silent main corridor. I passed Charlie the night porter on his way to the laboratory, carrying blood samples. He gave me a thumbs up and I smiled in return.

Arriving at the observation station, I recognised the nurse who had phoned as someone who generally knew her stuff. She took me to see a lady of about my mother's age. I noted the scar running down her breastbone and disappearing into her flowery cotton nightdress. I introduced myself and learned from her that she had a heart valve replaced a few days previously. I confirm this in the notes at the end of her bed. This was the first time we had met, as I worked on the male side of the unit by day, but covered problems on both male and female wards on alternate nights.

She was apologetic.

"Doctor, you didn't really need to get out of bed. I feel very well. It was only when I got up to use the toilet that I felt a sort of tightness at the back of my leg. Nurse Scott noticed me limping a little and didn't like the look of my ankle. I'm sorry to bother you at this time of night."

I reassured her it was no problem at all, as I examined her legs. There was no doubt the left calf muscle was tender and I was able to demonstrate what was known to me as Homan's sign. First I asked her to bend her knee, then with the knee bent, I flexed her foot up at the ankle joint. This caused a sharp pain in the belly of the gastrocnemius muscle in the calf above where it joined the Achilles tendon. This, and some swelling around her ankle confirmed that Avril Scott was right, Mrs. O'Leary had a clot in her lower leg - a deep venous thrombosis or DVT, brought on by prolonged bed rest. This was a potentially dangerous situation, as the clot may move up in the returning blood flow to settle in her lung, affecting her breathing and her heart. I explained the possible risk to her.

"This is not uncommon after all you've been through, Mrs. O'Leary," I reassured her. "Staff Nurse was quickly onto it, so I just need to start you on some treatment that'll dissolve the clot away at this early stage. We use a clot buster called Heparin which we give to you through your drip. Once that's running, you can get back to sleep."

"And maybe you can, too," she replied.

I set about writing a prescription, drew up the dose, and checked it with Nurse Scott. After a loading shot, I left a low dose infusion running until morning. I said goodbye to everyone, refused an offer of tea and headed for bed. I had been up for well over an hour. Back in my room, I ignored the overbearing heat again and crashed out.

All too soon, it was time for a shower, a shave and a bowl of cornflakes. Then back to the ward.

Now, I stood in front of my boss, rather shaken by his aggressive statement that I was in the shit.

"If you say so," I attempted to reply.

Ignoring this, he continued, "You have given an intravenous anticoagulant to one of my patients, for whom I had already prescribed an oral agent to thin her blood."

Remaining silent, I tried to think clearly. Had I made a terrible mistake?

"As long as you recognise you are in shit then maybe you can get this sorted out. I have to get to the operating theatre."

He abruptly left the room, as I was trying to tell him I would consult a haematologist for advice.

I went immediately to see Mrs. O'Leary, a dread in the pit of my stomach. She was in good spirits, smiled when she saw me, and told me she thought her leg might be a little easier. I told her that another specialist would soon be along to reassess her treatment.

The ward sister was sympathetic, and expressed her view that there had not been any harm done, but she had stopped the Heparin as instructed by the surgeon.

My phone call caught the Professor of Haematology, who had just reached her office. She agreed to come immediately and review the situation.

I awaited her verdict anxiously. She was unruffled and businesslike. She looked at me over her glasses.

"The thing is, your lady indeed has a DVT. I'm sure of that and the surgeon agrees. She was on oral Warfarin, but clearly it did not prevent a thrombosis forming in the leg. The correct course of action is to introduce intravenous Heparin which is inevitably an effective treatment. Oral Warfarin is more useful as a preventative measure than it is as a treatment once a thrombosis has developed. We will restart the Heparin infusion and I will monitor Mrs. O'Leary's blood results and keep in touch."

As she wrote all this in the patient notes, I felt like hugging her, such was my relief, but there had been enough unprofessional behaviour for one morning. I thanked her gratefully as she handed me the clinical folder. She gave sister a smile, and with a reassuring nod and a wink she left.

By then I really needed that cup of tea. The ward domestic already had the kettle boiled. As I sipped the brew, I reflected that the heroics and glamour of surgery had an undoubted appeal, but I was not sure I had the right macho temperament for it.

General surgery: poetic justice

"I've had an urgent request to assess a young man in Accident and Emergency" Peter, my new surgical registrar informed me as we walked briskly up the hospital corridor. "Bizarrely, he has been shot in the testicles from a passing car."

"Wow! That sounds bloody nasty. I was once struck there by a cricket ball, and it almost crippled me. I can't imagine what it would be like to be hit by a bullet."

We entered the patient's cubicle. The victim was in some distress, despite having received an injection of a strong analgesic. His groin area was covered by a sterile surgical drape, under which was an ice-cold dressing. Peter carefully peeled this away and we stared at the bruised and swollen organs. My own testicular muscles contracted involuntarily drawing them protectively upwards. Sympathetically, we asked what exactly had happened. He told us that he was standing outside a pub, smoking a cigarette, when someone in a passing car fired an automatic weapon at him.I considered that he was relatively lucky, after all, having escaped alive.

Gentle palpation suggested the testicles were probably intact, which gave some reassurance to the patient. When we stepped into the corridor, the staff nurse, who had stayed tactfully in the background, asked if we had examined the young man's trousers and underpants. Mystified, we admitted we had not thought to do so. A minute later she reappeared with the clothing and showed us the burnt and discoloured underpants and a pair of trousers with a single hole torn through the cloth in the rear upper thigh area. She looked at us expectantly.

"Well, what's your conclusion? You can see there is only one hole in the trousers."

At once we realised what she was suggesting.

"You think he had a gun, pushed it inside the front of his pants and it went off? " asked Peter. "A victim of poetic justice, rather than a passing gunman?"

She nodded grimly.

Unusual deposits

As I have mentioned, each general surgery ward in the hospital took turns to accept a day's surgical emergencies on a rotating basis. When a potential surgical problem arrived in casualty, they were vetted by the staff there and the ward on "take in" then contacted. The registrar would decide which patients needed admitting for potential surgical intervention. I often accompanied him (there were no female surgical registrars) to casualty and wrote up a detailed case history - either there, or when the person arrived in the ward. I then arranged any of the blood tests or investigations that were required. Junior doctors tended to learn a lot from this close working partnership, since registrars were either working towards, or had just completed, a higher medical or surgical qualification and were happy to display their knowledge.

Consultant surgeons were a little more remote from the junior house officers and not always so keen to teach. They had a wide range of personalities. I worked with one who rarely spoke but hummed, or quietly whistled hymns, while examining and reviewing patients, and when reading or writing up their notes. I would stand by, ignored, and have to check on what he had written later, to determine if there was anything I needed to do. I doubt he ever knew my name. At the opposite end of the spectrum was a handsome, charismatic and skilful surgeon on whom both female patients and nursing staff fawned. He apparently had a beautiful wife and eight children - but more importantly to me, he enjoyed teaching his juniors and was always readily available for advice.

The routine general surgery patients in my unit did not always have life threatening conditions. Rather, they suffered with ones that made their life miserable: Haemorrhoids, gallstones, duodenal or gastric ulcers. Some had more serious complaints, bowel and gastric cancer, or bowel diseases such as ulcerative colitis or Crohn's disease, both of which cause chronic diarrhoea and debility. Since my early days as a doctor, some of these problems have become more effectively managed by medical treatments. The advent of drugs known as proton pump inhibitors, which dramatically reduce stomach acid production, and the antibiotic eradication of certain bacteria in the stomach, can prevent and cure ulcers. A greater understanding of inflammatory bowel disease has led to treatments which alter underlying immunological factors. Many acute conditions such as appendicitis, of course, still generally require urgent surgery.

There were lighter moments to the work, such as one patient who was asked to return after surgery with a sample of his bowel motion. He did so, delivering a perfectly formed turd, which he had managed to deposit in a narrow-necked glass milk bottle. With some glee, we sent it on to the laboratory wondering how they might retrieve the contents for analysis. On another occasion, a post-vasectomy patient left a brown paper envelope with a follow-up sperm sample inside. No nurse would touch it. I was summoned to explain, again, the leaflet he had received, but possibly not read, and to provide him with a more appropriate receptacle.

Tragedy, however, was never far away.

The Abercorn Restaurant bomb

On the first Saturday in March 1972, an IRA bomb exploded in a packed Belfast city-centre restaurant. I was just one month into my surgical attachments.

As the House Officer on duty for my ward that weekend, I was relaxing in the doctor's On Call room with a few colleagues when the phone rang. The person who answered responded with only a few short words before turning and calling above the noise of the television, "There's been a major bomb explosion downtown and they need everyone to get to casualty now!"

We all rushed out of the room, the sports results forgotten.

I knew the target well, The Abercorn Restaurant and Bar. It was an extremely popular venue with weekend shoppers for lunch or coffee and a snack. The bomb was left under a table to the rear. When it detonated, the blast ripped through the crowded cafe, killing two young women, one of whom was a radiographer in our hospital. In all, 130 customers and staff were injured, some horrifically. The shock wave from the explosion had spread with enormous force under the tables, resulting in several people, including two sisters, losing limbs.

When I reached the emergency department, the victims were just beginning to arrive in ambulances. A senior surgical registrar and the staff nurse in charge were attempting to triage the casualties. The treatment cubicles were cleared of people with minor complaints in order to accommodate the seriously injured. The number of casualties and severity of many of the injuries were beyond anything I had experienced before. Most arrivals were filthy from the debris of the explosion in which they had been caught. It was not a time for panic, we just had to start trying to help stabilise those worst injured. In the midst of the frantic activity and noise, I was directed to a cubicle where the patient was unconscious and in severe shock due to major trauma and blood loss. I was instructed to get an intravenous line in place in order to transfuse blood and plasma to support their circulation. I immediately set about placing a needle into a vein in the arm, but the blood pressure was so low that the vessels were collapsed and shut down. I opted to cut down to a large leg vein with a scalpel but, on uncovering the legs, I realised the damage to the lower limbs was so severe that this was not an option. As a fear that I was going to lose my patient began to grip me, a senior obstetrician I recognised appeared through the curtains. He was one of the many people who came from all over the hospital, and from home, to help. He rapidly recognised my dilemma, shouted to me to stay calm and disappeared through the curtains. Almost immediately he reappeared with a chunky red hardback book entitled, *Pye's Surgical Handicraft*.

"We may need to cut down to the large subclavian vein, where it travels under the collar bone," he said. We rapidly looked at the diagram and instructions. As his deep cut was made with a scalpel blade, I retracted the skin to expose the vessel.

Shortly a line was sutured in place, and I was left again, now with a nurse, to connect up the bag of O negative blood. This blood type is known as the universal donor, as it can be given to people with any of the various blood groups, in an emergency. We placed a blood pressure cuff around the bag, gradually inflating it to speed up the delivery. The victim's blood pressure slowly started to climb before we attached a second unit.

While some of the details from that hectic day are vague now, I can still picture that red book. I know my patient had been given morphine and was probably deeply unconscious throughout these events. I hope so.

I have a brief glimpse in my mind's eye of passing a surgeon, as I moved to another cubicle. He was demanding a vial of morphine from a nurse. She seemed to have been tasked to make sure the dispensing of dangerous opioid drugs was properly documented and was asking for his signature, briefly delaying its release.

"To hell with the DDA record book," he was shouting in frustration.

I spent a considerable time during the next few hours suturing lacerations or splinting broken limbs, working with junior colleagues and nurses, some with no casualty experience, who were calming terrified individuals while cleaning and dressing their wounds.

Late in the day, I was in theatre where, by now, it was the less critically injured who were being operated on.

The patient with whom I was now involved had a wooden chair leg speared right through the thigh, but seemed remarkably comfortable due to the effect of strong analgesics. In order to induce anaesthesia, a muscle relaxant is always administered to stop the patient breathing, so that the mechanical ventilator can take over.

When the now-anaesthetised patient was moved onto the operating table, to my amazement, the chair leg fell to the floor. The relaxant drug had stopped the quadriceps muscle from spasming, suddenly releasing it. There was, of course still, a nasty and penetrating track to be cleaned and treated.

In the early hours of Sunday morning, when the last operation was finished and casualty at last cleared, the senior surgeon of the day turned to some of us to ask who held the key to the junior doctor's bar.

"I want to meet all of you there in 10 minutes for a short debrief."

When he arrived, he thanked us all for our work.

"I know you have seen things today which I hope you never see again, and I know you probably feel exhausted. You may, however, have trouble getting to sleep, so I am prescribing a stiff drink all round. So, each of you will have a brandy or whisky, on me." He spent the next 20 minutes making sure he had spoken to each one of us personally.

It was probably the nearest thing to counselling we ever had.

Despite the widespread public revulsion at this incident, in which the lives of innocent people were again lost, and those of many others changed forever, another bomb was detonated in the city centre only a few weeks later, in a busy area, at lunch hour. This time seven people were killed and around 150 injured.

Not long afterwards, on Easter Sunday, I sat in church and heard prayers offered up for the victims of these tragedies, and for the doctors and nurses who attended them. I thought then, as I do now, that of all the professionals involved, it was the ambulance crews who had the most traumatic experiences. They rarely had the chance to see again, the people they had rescued. They transported not just the injured and the dying but also the dead. They saw the mutilation caused by bombs at first hand, a horror from which the perpetrators escaped.

A last chance

Alongside such events, routine surgery carried on in my unit and, on occasions, I enjoyed the opportunity to assist in the operating theatre, usually with one surgeon who shared my relatively short stature.

In June, the surgery finals examination again took place in our ward. It seemed hard to believe a year had passed since I had been a candidate myself. The consultants had drawn up a list of suitable patients and obtained their consent to take part. I was in the ward early, making sure that the examiner would have a brief clinical summary for each.

On the list of candidates was a student who was said to be an American, and who had already failed to pass on several previous attempts at the examination He was considered to be rather eccentric. For example, it was believed that he now disdained using standard undergraduate textbooks, preferring to read articles in the medical journals to refine his knowledge. He was to be seen intermittently around the hospital, walking with a determined elongated stride, or spotted studying in the depths of the library. He seemed not to socialise with any other students. Apparently he performed well when, rarely, he attended a teaching session. An unsubstantiated and unlikely rumour suggested he might be failing deliberately, in order to avoid being drafted to Vietnam, where the war still raged. My boss was determined he should be given one final opportunity to suceed if it was at all possible.

This year, his main case for diagnosis was a man who had lost a considerable amount of weight and had been passing blood with his bowel motions. If a student performed a rectal examination, he would easily detect a palpable tumour. In order to pass the examination, all they had to do was identify this growth. Each student was allowed an hour with a patient. With 10 minutes remaining, the examining consultant asked me if the candidate had requested the rectal examination tray which contained gloves, lubricant, and wipes. He had not.

I was told to go and ask him if there was anything he needed. He reassured me there was nothing. It was then suggested I might return and ask if he would like to have the PR (per rectum) examination tray, as he now had only five minutes left. Again, he thanked me with a, "No, thank you". This sort of unbidden prompting was highly irregular, and could not happen today. Nevertheless, I was then instructed to bring the tray and silently set it on the patient's bed. It remained there untouched and our friend, who unsurprisingly did not suggest the correct diagnosis, failed again. The university rules had changed around this time, so that only a limited number of attempts at the final exam were permitted. I do not think this young man ever graduated. For years, I wondered what drove him, and what his demons really were. Some individuals who are seduced by the glamour and kudos of medicine in the media, find they are unable to cope with its demands, responsibilities and the reality of death and suffering. I hope he found fulfilment elsewhere.

Farewell

At the end of July, I finished what had turned out, overall, to have been a fulfilling, if at times tense and challenging year as a Junior House Officer. Completing the clinical training qualified me for full registration as a doctor with the General Medical Council. Throughout that last month, I was torn in deciding between the specialties I should choose for my next post, since it would probably determine my ultimate career path.

I had spent a year doing something I had long dreamed of. The dream was of treating ill people and ultimately saving lives. Sadly, I was faced repeatedly throughout that year by the fact that a few of my countrymen were prepared to do the opposite. Indeed, just ten days before the end of my post, on 21 July, 1972, 20 bombs exploded in Belfast in the space of 90 minutes. Nine people were killed and over 100 injured. That day became known as Bloody Friday.

Over the previous 12 months, there had been casualties from all sides of this conflict, including some whose lives I had helped to save. On occasions, the antagonists ended up only metres apart in the same ward, receiving the same dedicated care from nurses, some of whom had battled to reach work through the dangers these individuals helped to create.

In the casualty department, I had seen some of the worst things men could do. But the place where I had seen the best of humanity and best hope for the future was the Children's Hospital. The children there were my heroes, showing courage in the face of an enemy they did not understand or deserve, with loving parents suppressing their own anguish, to allay their little one's distress and pain

78

I had, inevitably developed an admiration for the surgeons I encountered who practised their craft with skill, even when under stress or faced with the need to take a risk to save a life - but not perhaps for the arrogance and hubris of a select few. As a student there was always an attraction in imagining becoming a part of the glamorous media portrayal of surgery, but this had faded.

Equally, I was impressed by physician scientists who dissected complex cases, employing sharp minds to assess clinical facts, used laboratory tests and other investigations to logically reach a diagnosis and prescribe a successful treatment.

But along with many of these qualities I admired, I identified most with the kindness, empathy and altruism I saw in career paediatricians. I was drawn to the challenge of earning the trust of parents and children, of restoring health to young patients with all of their lives ahead of them, and who might have the potential to change the world. It was from these children I found my inspiration and vocation.

4. Joining the paediatric team

Appointed as a Senior House Officer (SHO) in Paediatrics, I returned to the ward which I knew as a student and a JHO. Rebecca had gone, her trachea repaired at a specialist unit. I heard that she could talk now, and had been back to visit a few times. She was full of stories about her life in the real world, no longer enthralled by the sight of the flames in a living room fireplace. Her delights were now in more normal childhood pastimes - playing outside, going to the park, or visiting cousins' houses.

Workload 1972

I now had the luxury of working what almost seemed a normal five-day week, only being required to be resident in the hospital one night in four, although also on every fourth weekend. It was a matter of professional pride to ensure each evening, when we handed over to the person on call for the night, that all routine ward work was complete. While this sometimes meant getting home well past an agreed dinner time, it helped each of us on the rota survive through busy evenings. When we were newly qualified Junior House Officers, we had all lived full time in the hospital because we worked alternate nights and weekends. Between Friday morning and Monday evening, this amounted to 80 continuous hours, with sleep snatched when (and if) things were quiet. JHOs worked on average more than 100 hours each week. As an SHO, this now dropped to around 70 hours. Of course, if a colleague was ill or on leave, the number of hours jumped back up proportionately.

I enjoyed, even loved, the paediatric work - looking after sick children in a team. As doctors we worked closely not only with nurses and other colleagues, but also with parents and grandparents. Inevitably families were totally committed to helping their children and each other through an illness, no matter how unpleasant or prolonged the treatment. The idea of specific visiting times, still standard practice in adult units, was obsolete here. Parents were the only people who spent more time in the hospital than junior doctors.

Nights and weekends were often hectic. My radio bleep would alert me that I was needed somewhere. A call to the hospital's switchboard operator would let me know exactly where. Next, I contacted the ward to find out what they needed me to do. As I sorted out the problem, the bleep often sounded again. The pattern repeated for hours, and so time flew by. Medical consultants were rarely seen out of hours, except perhaps in the Intensive Care Unit - although surgeons and anaesthetists came in for emergency operations.

The Accident and Emergency Department did not have a dedicated consultant and was staffed by Senior House Officers and Registrars. The latter, at least, had higher professional qualifications, and a few years training, but it was from the nurse in charge, still with the title "Sister," who had vast practical experience, that I learned most: how to set and plaster a broken arm, how to manage and terminate a seizure, how to recognise a non-accidental injury, and a great deal more.

More children attended the department between the hours of 5 p.m. and 9 p.m. than did between 9 a.m. and 5 p.m.. Mothers who had nursed an unwell child with a raised temperature during the day tended to panic as the long night approached. There was a belief in the local community that going to the hospital A&E meant their little ones would be seen by a proper "children's doctor". The reality was that the hospital employed experienced general practitioners to help staff the unit between 6 p.m. and 10 p.m. and at the busiest times at the weekend. This was to release the junior doctors to concentrate on ward work. From a life in family practice, these old hands had long ago acquired the skill I was now gradually developing; how to tell the difference between an unwell and a seriously ill child. Some had been paediatric registrars before changing careers. At least one was a little unorthodox in managing an overcrowded waiting area. He would stand on a chair and roar, "Hands up anyone who has already seen their GP today?" Many of those sitting on the benches would look confused, some uncertain raised an arm.

"Anyone who has not consulted their family doctor should leave at once and do so now."

He would then step down and return to the treatment area. On one such occasion, I noted Sister intercepting the few parents and children as they were getting up to leave and performing a discrete triage, advising any patient with more than a minor complaint that they must stay.

At night, and for most of the weekend, there were only four doctors in the hospital, which had six wards. One SHO looked after the medical wards and patients, while another was responsible for the surgical side. Registrars were next in seniority, but they were not always on site. The surgical registrar, for instance, had responsibilities not only in our hospital, but also for inpatient paediatric problems and emergencies at the District General Hospital, 10 miles away. Also on our site was the maternity hospital which had a special care baby unit (SCBU). If a premature baby in the SCBU became unwell, the paediatric registrar would be summoned. If there was an emergency caesarean section out of hours, they'd be crash-called to be on hand when the baby was delivered. If all was quiet, the registrar might get an hour or two at home (if it was nearby) returning around 10 p.m., when together we would review the newly-admitted patients, those who were seriously ill, or any about whom I wanted advice. I would then walk the 200-or-so metres to the maternity unit to check on the babies there, hoping that I might spend most of the night in the on-call bedroom, while the registrar stayed in the children's hospital.

Rhesus babies

As the SHO, I always had one final task each night before any sleep might be possible. This was checking the severity of jaundice in our Rhesus babies. Just judging how yellow they had become was not enough. A blood test to measure the level of bilirubin, the substance which causes jaundice,was required. This involved what we called a heel stab; a careful needle prick in the soft part of the baby's heel to produce a tiny bead of blood This was then sent off to the duty biochemist. Bilirubin is released when red blood cells are broken down.

Rhesus babies inherit the Rhesus (D) blood group from their father but their mothers are Rhesus negative. On the surface of these babies' red cells is the Rhesus D antigen, so they too are designated Rhesus positive. The maternal red cells have no D antigen, they are Rhesus negative.

During any pregnancy a few foetal blood cells cross the placenta and enter the mother's blood stream. A rhesus negative mother's immune system will recognise 'foreign' Rhesus positive blood in her circulation, and form antibodies against them. These destroy the 'foreign' red cells.

The initial reaction is generally too weak to cause a problem. This usually happens with a first pregnancy or perhaps a miscarriage. However, the mother is now sensitised to recognise and react to any future encounter with Rhesus positive blood.

On a second such pregnancy, the numerous antibodies created easily cross back through the placenta and damage the baby's red blood cells. This results in the release of the bilirubin pigment. Before birth, the bilirubin crosses back across the placenta and is safely metabolised by the mother. After delivery however there is continued release of bilirubin, as the maternal antibodies persist for some time in the child's circulation. The newborn's immature liver has a limited capacity to neutralise the bilirubin. Jaundice therefore develops after birth, and eventually, a high level of bilirubin may be reached, when there is a risk of it entering and damaging the baby's brain.

My first response to a rising level was to prescribe phototherapy, a treatment not unlike using a sunbed. This utilised a specific wavelength of blue light, which fortunately has the property of breaking down bilirubin in the skin. The baby was nursed naked under the light with its eyes protected. Before initiating this treatment, I would sit down with the mother, and hopefully the father, to explain all the possible protective actions which might be required, and make sure the potential risks were understood. Of course, shortly after giving birth is not the ideal time to be receiving worrying news.

If the bilirubin reached a critical level, I would be faced with two or three tiring hours carrying out an exchange blood transfusion. This replaces most of the baby's blood with Rhesus negative donor blood, and simultaneously removes bilirubin from the circulation. To perform this, I removed the clamp from the cut umbilical chord and dissected out the vessels in the stump. Before birth these vessels carried the baby's blood to and from the placenta. I was then able to introduce a venous cannula. Through this, double the baby's total blood volume would be gradually removed, 10 millilitres at a time, and replaced each time by freshly donated, safe rhesus negative blood. Throughout the delicate procedure, I was always assisted by a midwife or nurse. We were acutely aware that if the procedure was performed too rapidly, it might cause the infant's blood sugar to fall, or precipitate heart failure. Both the blood sugar levels and heart activity were constantly monitored. The monotonous regular bleep of the cardiac monitor, while reassuring, could be soporific unless there was a sudden change in the rhythm. A strong coffee and a visit to the toilet before starting was wise. By the end, with a stiff neck and shoulders, my own blood sugar level was likely to be rather low. As the tension drained away, it was good to be able to report to the parents that all was well and any danger passed for now. Their baby was safe.

Today, an anti Rhesus antibody, derived from donated blood known as Anti D immunoglobulin is given to Rhesus negative mothers who are at risk of having Rhesus babies, early in and during pregnancy. This prevents the mother developing antibodies against Rhesus positive blood cells by destroying them before sensitisation can occur.

A sudden infant death

Despite only having three months of previous paediatric experience, I was occasionally the only doctor in the A&E Department on a weekend morning. Adventurous children trickled in after falls from trees, the tops of walls, down stairs, off bicycles; or with bumps and sprains suffered at school football matches and other sports. Sorting these problems out became routine, as were children presenting with vomiting, diarrhoea and minor respiratory complaints.

Harrowing events, such as what we then called a cot death, or dealing with the results of a major road traffic accident, however, left an indelible mark. Faced one Saturday morning with an apparently dead infant, my automatic reaction was to initiate full resuscitation procedures while calling for senior back up, suppressing the feeling in my heart that the child was beyond help. Like the parents, I hoped and prayed we might somehow get him back. They watched, clutching each other, as we worked frantically but to no avail. Thankfully my registrar and a consultant were there almost immediately and took over managing the tragic situation. Eventually I stood by, numb, listening to my senior colleague as he sat talking as kindly as possible to the couple, now beyond grief or comfort. How, I wondered, would he explain that the coroner must be informed, that the police and social services would become involved, and a post mortem performed? Other family members and a priest arrived. Several times, he repeated that such sudden deaths were rare; that often, as on that day, no cause was identified; and such tragedies were certainly no one's fault. After leaving the family alone for a time, we returned and he again explained that certain investigations were required by law, not because of any suspicions. I listened closely to how he gently explained and became choked as the baby lay motionless in the mother's arms. They were unaware of me, as I spoke my condolences and touched their shoulders before leaving, my eyes burning.

A sudden unexplained infant death is a devastating event for a family and shocking to nurses and doctors. While still the commonest cause of death in children under the age of one year, it was twice as common in the 1970s and is still not fully understood. One reason for the substantial fall in incidence was the discovery in the 1980s that laying babies to sleep on their backs, rather than on their tummies, was by far the safest position. This recommendation was initially greeted by scepticism - particularly, in my experience, by grandmothers - but the subsequent drop in numbers confirmed the wise advice promoted by the public health "Back to Sleep" campaign.

An innocent inquiry

I walked slowly back to my ward that morning knowing that, inevitably, there would be routine but essential tasks to be performed. These demands, the shared sorrow and mutual support from the team, and the background noise of the small children made it possible to continue with the day's essential work.

Simple conversations with my patients could sometimes brighten the darkest day and recharge depleted emotional batteries.

"Where has your moustache gone?" a little boy inquired a short time later, staring intently at my face as I examined his chest. He had been admitted for investigations of a chronic cough and loss of weight just a few days before, when I had met him and his family for the first time. He was still fascinated by his new surroundings and especially the ward's large fish tank.

"I don't actually have a moustache," I replied, wondering why he had asked. It made me remember my one abortive attempt at growing a moustache as a student, which sadly only invited derision from my mates.

"Yes, you do!', he shouted, bouncing on the bed, as his mother tried to calm and distract him.

He leaned in, bringing his laughing face even closer to mine, and pointed.

"It's up your nose!" he announced triumphantly.

Meningitis

Early on another morning, a distressed young woman came running into the emergency department carrying a baby wrapped in a cot blanket. Our experienced casualty sister assessed the situation at a glance and took control. She reached out, took the baby from the girl's arms and briskly walked the few steps to the resuscitation room, calling my name as she went. As I hurried to join her, she gently laid the baby on the examination couch. I would remember forever the strange, weak, high-pitched cry coming from the child. We removed his clothes and recognised the blotchy purple rash and red blood coloured spots on his skin. We both immediately knew the cause: Meningococcal meningitis and septicaemia. I turned to a staff nurse who had just found a seat for the tear-stained mother.

"Put an urgent call out for the senior registrar, and quickly," I said.

The parents had thought the baby was a little out of sorts at bedtime the previous evening. During the night, he was restless and reluctant to feed. On waking in the morning, he had a runny nose and felt a little hot. They phoned to speak to their family doctor. He had not yet arrived at his surgery. They gave their little boy a cool bath while they waited to contact him again for advice. It was then that they noticed a rash like little red pin pricks on his tummy. As his mum dried and dressed him, she realised the rash had spread to his legs and bottom. The spots were bigger. They waited no longer but immediately set off by car for the children's hospital, which was only a few minute's drive away. On the short journey, his mum noticed several times that his eyes seemed to be rolling. By the time they arrived, she was terrified because she could get little response from her baby. She jumped out of the car with the child and left his dad to get parked.

I examined him as calmly as I could, with fear gripping my heart. Pallor, a rapid but weak pulse and low blood pressure confirmed he was in septic shock. Senior help was with me almost immediately. Intravenous infusions of plasma improved his circulation and oxygen was administered by facemask as we rushed him to the paediatric intensive care unit (PICU) across the corridor. The parents gave permission for a lumbar puncture to be performed and blood samples were also taken for analysis and culture. He received a combination of three antibiotics intravenously. Shortly after 9 a.m. his airway was intubated, and supportive mechanical respiratory ventilation commenced. He was now on full life support.

I spoke to the shocked parents as the PICU team worked with him. I explained about the various monitors and tubes now in place, in an attempt to lessen the shock when they went in to see their little boy. I confirmed that the baby was critically ill, but stable, and explained the consultant was waiting to speak to them inside the unit.

I returned to the emergency department, where a queue of patients was waiting to be seen.

At midday the baby's heart stopped.

He responded to resuscitation initially but, five hours later, he suffered a further cardiac arrest from which he did not recover. All that was left to do was try to comfort his mother and father, now surrounded by their family. My final task that day was to arrange for each to have protective antibiotics to eradicate any of the bacteria they might be harbouring.

Although I had learnt, as a student, about how devastating a meningococcal infection could be, I was still shocked by this first-hand experience of its rapid progress. An otherwise healthy baby had died in less than 24 hours, despite the rapid action of his parents, and every effort being made to save him at a major children's hospital.

In the following months, I was to see over 40 children with meningococcal infections. Although not all developed the fulminant form of the disease, there were seven who died. There were four or five times as many cases that year than usual, most in infants and children under the age of two. The attrition rate had an enormous impact on me. On several occasions, I had discussions about the upsurge in cases and the number of deaths with my senior colleagues. Professor Carré, my boss, encouraged me to collect data about the outbreak in order to learn all I could about the condition. He suggested I write about my experience in the local medical journal, to inform others. The result was my first scientific publication.

It appeared to me then, that once the bacteria entered the bloodstream, causing a septicaemia (often called sepsis today), the chances of recovery became extremely slim. In light of this, preventing these infections seemed to be the best option, if lives were to be saved.

The spectre of meningococcal disease determined our approach to any unwell or drowsy infant presenting with an unexplained fever or a seizure. On each one, we performed a lumbar puncture under sterile conditions, inserting a needle between two vertebrae, low down the baby's spine, to obtain a sample of cerebrospinal fluid (CSF). I had become quite adept at this procedure, which is less commonly performed today thanks to the early administration of broad-spectrum antibiotics - an approach which may be reviewed due to the increase in antibiotic resistance. The organism's DNA can now also be detected by molecular biological techniques in blood and spinal fluid.

There are several types or subgroups of the meningococcal bacteria. The most common then was group C. A vaccine against this became available in the US a few years later, in 1975, but it was found to be relatively ineffective in the most vulnerable age group: Infants and children under the age of two. It was 15 years before this vaccine was routinely given to children in the UK. Within a few years, the number of infections with group C fell to almost zero in all ages. However, meningococcal disease continued to be a killer as group B organisms became the most prevalent cause. Eventually, for the first time, in 2015 all babies in the UK were vaccinated against meningococcus B strain from the age of 2 months.

In 2010, out of the blue, I received a letter from a family in Strabane.

"You will not remember us, or our son Ronan. You and your team treated him on 12th January, 1993 for meningococcal septicaemia. His dad and I always said that if he ever got married, we would love to have you at the wedding. He is a lovely lad and we love him very much.

Attracta and Ronnie Johnstone."

I was delighted to attend the wedding with my wife - and delighted to meet Ronan again, alongside his beautiful bride. I was delighted most of all to hear the hilarious stories his best man told at the reception afterwards, confirming Ronan was one of the fortunate victims who came through unscathed. Ten percent of survivors have major disabilities, including amputations, brain injury and deafness. Thirty per cent have significant but less serious after effects.

Hopefully, the introduction of effective vaccines against all the strains of this potentially lethal organism, and their worldwide use, will make such infections and its complications a rarity.

When I read about vaccine deniers in the modern era, I am appalled and saddened. Those of us who saw the devastating effects not just of meningococcal disease, but also of measles and other childhood infections, dread the thought of turning back the clock.

The experience of tracking the meningococcal meningitis outbreak brought me face to face with the reality of death in childhood. In the 1970s, around 50 children in every 100,000, between the ages of one and 15, died. This number has fallen to single figures in the twenty-first century (7 out of every 100,000 in 2021). While the outlook for many serious and chronic conditions has significantly improved over the years, any young life lost remains a devastating event. When such a death is sudden or unexpected, as with a "cot death" (SIDS) or as a result of a traffic or other accident, there is a terrible and lasting impact on a family.

Gradually, I would come to realise the limitations of heroic hospital treatment in some of these situations. In fact, preventative measures were, and are, the better way to avert some such heartaches - whether it's changing the position in which babies are put down to sleep, compulsory seat belts and child restraints in cars, or routine vaccination against infection.

There was little time, as a junior doctor, to consider or recognise the limited support for bereaved parents, nor to understand that they would feel their loss for the rest of their lives.

Thankfully, on most days, the pleasure of seeing the vast majority of our patients bouncing back to health helped us cope at a personal level and more than offset the busy days and long nights.

5. Important discoveries

During my early time in paediatrics, I made two or three major personal discoveries. The first, and most important, I realised I had fallen in love.

The second was that as a couple, we were unlikely to be able to afford a house with our limited assets and current salaries. Certainly not one with the potential to be a family home. I was loath to consider renting, which might be the alternative option today.

The third was that I was perhaps not as clever as I had imagined.

Romance

At the height of the troubles, pubs became risky places to spend an evening in West Belfast - or, indeed, any part of the city. They were repeatedly targets for gun attacks and bombs. Outside the hospital, sporadic rioting could suddenly flare. Security roadblocks were common. To avoid travelling too far for entertainment, medical students and junior staff who lived in the hospital complex, developed a unique, but safe, internal social life. In this respect, at least, our situation was not unlike that in various embattled areas of the city, where local people also only mixed with those they knew and strangers were understandably viewed with suspicion.

One winter evening, I was enjoying one of the parties we regularly organised in the hospital residential quarters. They boasted a small bar, furnished with a variety of comfortable, well worn, somewhat-beer-stained armchairs and sofas. Across the dimly lit room, I recognised an attractive young woman whose brown eyes were almost hidden behind a long fringe of shiny dark hair. She was a nurse I'd noticed working efficiently in one of the wards, her good humour cheering up the patients. I was attracted then - as I am now - by this girl who was having an enjoyable time with her friends, seemingly oblivious of the available male talent. I was unaware that these girls hunted in a pack. As the disco music blasted out from a makeshift audio system, I managed to have a couple of dances with her, before being called on to take my turn serving at the bar. I felt I was making an impression and enlisted the help of my friend, Kenny.

"I really fancy my chances with that girl. Would you keep an eye out for her, until I finish my stint at the bar?"

I left him chatting to her and her friends. By the time I had handed over to the next person on the bar roster, they had all vanished.

"What happened?", I asked Kenny.

"I think they got bored and went home."

Clearly, my interest had not been reciprocated.

With some difficulty I tracked Anne down some months later and invited her gang to another party, this time organised in the maternity hospital residence. While chatting to her about paediatrics, I offered to take her to see the premature babies in our neonatal unit, which was in the same building. This turned out to be a more successful idea than I had anticipated and I began to hope that, at the very least, I had fired a spark of interest. My recollection is that, with the night sister's permission, we donned sterile gowns and overshoes and briefly toured the incubators, gazing with awe at the tiny infants inside. As we walked back in the subdued night lighting along the quiet hospital corridor, I suggested we might meet up again the following weekend for a meal, or something more interesting. She unhelpfully informed me this wouldn't be possible as she was travelling to her home, some 60 miles away on the north coast. Despite it dawning on me that it was perhaps only the babies she was attracted to, I did not give up my pursuit and suggested I could drive her there.

Suddenly, there was a flicker of interest.

"Oh, you have a car?"

This happily clinched the date, perhaps because it saved a long train journey, not to mention the fare. To be fair, she was unaware of how unreliable my elderly Mini was.

One evening, some time later, as I left Anne back to her flat - which was in a tower block at the rear of the hospital - there was a burst of gunfire as we got out of the car. We threw ourselves to the ground beside the car and lay together until the shooting stopped, before making a dash for the entrance. Perhaps it was inevitable that we became close friends.

As I got to know Anne better, I was captivated by her bubbly personality, which had the ability to brighten not only her patient's days but, now, also mine. It was not long before I began to think this was a girl I might marry one day. Most of my colleagues were not quite ready for this sort of commitment but when I confided in John, one of my best friends, he said, "Just do it, go ahead and ask her!" He had already recognised I was what he considered "a lost cause".

The salary for junior doctors in the 1970s was not generous. There was no extra pay for weekend or night time work, just a basic salary of around £80 per month after tax deduction, for a working week of up to 80 hours. Gaps in the hospital's rota, caused by illness or unfilled posts, were covered for no extra remuneration by the remaining members of a junior team. Management did not consider this practice unreasonable, considering neither the risk to patient safety, nor the possible effect on employees' wellbeing. Initially, neither did we. For a month as a house surgeon in my first year, I covered two jobs. I was paired with a colleague to look after 50 or 60 patients across two wards until, unfortunately, my friend developed chicken pox and was sent off on sick leave. It did not occur to me to question such extra demands. I was living my dream job and, at that age, could tolerate the long hours, both physically and emotionally. As the most junior doctors, we worked and lived together in a mutually supportive environment. We took it for granted that our responsibility to our patients was the priority and that, to this end, we would naturally help each other, sharing advice, experiences and practical help. At least we did not have the millstone of student debt hanging around our necks, as is common today.

Moonlighting

By the time Anne and I fixed a date for our wedding, a year or two later, my meagre savings were still insufficient to secure a mortgage on any size of property.

Around this time, a more senior trainee doctor identified a market for short locum positions in general practice in the NHS. It was not uncommon then for newly qualified doctors to go straight into practice soon after having completed their trainee hospital house jobs (internships), which entitled them to become fully registered with the General Medical Council. Many family doctors had few, if any, junior partners, so that illness and holidays presented a problem in maintaining the continuity of their daily round of house calls, surgeries, and emergency night cover. He developed an unofficial locum supply agency for local family doctors who occasionally needed reliable stand-ins. Gradually, he compiled a list of junior hospital doctors willing to provide the cover. In reality, this was a vital service in the tense area of the city around the hospital. The payment for a three-hour surgery session paid almost as much as a couple of days of long hours in the hospital. He was careful in vetting people for this lucrative sideline, only offering opportunities to those he judged to be academically competent and who reportedly had reliable clinical skills and sound judgement. He provided brief tutorials and advice on problems likely to be encountered, including safe drug prescribing, supplemented by a mini drug formulary which he had developed.

I received a call one lunchtime at the end of a busy week, as I was about to have a rare and hard-earned half day's leave. I was almost flattered when he asked if I was interested in filling in that evening for a local doctor who was faced by an unforeseen family crisis. I was doubtful, but eager to help a colleague out of a predicament. I admit that when he quoted the going rate for the session, I agreed with only a little hesitation.

So began a new, invaluable, if unorthodox, phase of my medical education.

I arrived at the address I had been given, 10 or 15 minutes before the evening walk-in surgery was due to start. An elderly caretaker was waiting to unlock the dilapidated premises on the ground floor of a residential block in a deprived area close to the hospital. There was no sign of any other staff, no receptionist or nurse. This turned out to be a satellite surgery of a large practice based a mile or so away. It seemed I would be on my own, armed with my stethoscope, my large medical textbook and a copy of the British National Formulary of approved prescription drugs, which I had the foresight to bring along. The caretaker confirmed my suspicions that no other help was forthcoming and asked that I should make sure the door was locked if I was leaving before 7.30 p.m., at which time he would call back. He left and I carried out a brief exploration of the premises before patients began to appear and occupy the 12 sturdy, hard-backed chairs in the waiting area. There were various posters displayed on the walls relating to vaccinations and other services available on the NHS. Most looked, like the seats, as if they had been there for many years. There was, of course, a selection of old, well-thumbed magazines on a small coffee table in the centre of the room. A door in one corner was labelled Toilet. I did not venture inside.

Beyond this was the consultation room, which a plastic sign identified rather grandly as the "Doctor's Surgery". All the walls were painted a depressing, dull magnolia. My room was furnished with three chairs and an impressive desk. This was positioned under the one opaque security glass window, so that the doctor sitting there had some natural light, fortunately boosted at this time of evening by an angle poise lamp. I reckoned that, by sitting sideways to the desk, it was just possible to see the person entering through the door opposite. The whole place had a musty air of neglect. Two of the office's side walls were obscured by filing cabinets and high cupboards. The cabinets, I discovered, contained patients' files in reasonable alphabetical order. Curious, I made the mistake of opening some of the cupboards. From one, I was showered by a cascade of old drug starter packs and brochures, left by pharmaceutical company representatives, probably stuffed in there in the hope that one day they might come in useful. I had just managed to shove these back inside when there was a knock at the door to announce the first patient.

" Come in," I called with some trepidation.

A young woman entered looking rather anxious, yet determined. I introduced myself, asked her name and tried to locate her record in the basic filing system. Relieved to retrieve this successfully, I sat down facing her and asked how I could help. She came straight to the point.

"Do you do pregnancy tests here?" she asked. I stuttered an explanation that I was only filling in for the evening and would have to check. I went to the waiting room and confirmed again that no receptionist had arrived. Then, thankful that at least I had reconnoitred the contents of the cupboards, I recovered from one of them a couple of urine sample bottles. This was long before the advent of home pregnancy tests, where simply urinating on a stick can detect the presence of the hormone human chorionic gonadotropin (hGC), giving a positive result.

"One of these needs to be filled and brought in first thing on Monday morning," I explained, handing them over, since I had no idea how I might dispatch it to the hospital laboratory - which was unlikely to carry out such tests at that time of the evening anyway. I added it would probably take 48 hours for the result to come back. I started to make a note in the woman's file. At this point I discovered from previous entries she had been prescribed the contraceptive pill regularly, and realised I had not discussed her obstetric history.

"I see you are on the pill," I said. She nodded.

"So why do you think you might be pregnant?"

She disclosed that she had missed two menstrual periods and her breasts felt as they had during her previous three pregnancies.

"Did you ever miss taking the tablets?" I asked quietly. She was definite she had not.

To emphasise this, she added that, on one recent week when the family were staying at the seaside, she'd forgotten to bring her contraceptives and, rather than miss any pills, borrowed some from a friend in the next caravan.

I looked at her sympathetically, trying not to show what I was thinking. I checked the name of the contraceptive she was prescribed. It was an "everyday" type, which provided 28 tablets in a foil package, each labelled with the days of the week. Of these, 21 would contain a hormone which prevents ovulation, and seven would be blank tablets containing no medication . After seven days of taking the blanks, a light menstrual bleed is usually precipitated. I still wonder which of these two types she had obtained from her neighbour. If she'd borrowed blank tablets, it was likely she was pregnant.

I was receiving a practical lesson in the importance of making sure a patient understands their medication. I tried to explain gently what I suspected - and established that she had shared her suspicion with her husband. Before she left with the sample bottles in her handbag, I gave her my best wishes for whatever news her doctor would have on her next visit.

The next couple of hours raced past. Most of the problems were straightforward. I prescribed nonstop; antibiotics for respiratory infections, bronchodilators to reverse the wheeze of asthma, cough remedies, (from the provided list, since we did not use these relatively ineffective syrups in hospital), and pain killers for arthritis. I listened to people's complaints and problems as patiently as I could, while occasionally wondering how many others were waiting to be seen. I continued pulling and replacing patient's notes, as each one entered and left. The file for one overweight elderly lady proved to be missing. She had come to have her prescription for "heart tablets" renewed. She could not name them so I attempted to deduce from her description as to what these might be. I was fairly sure she was taking a diuretic to increase urine output and reduce fluid accumulation which might overload her heart. The clue was in her explanation that if she missed these her ankles would swell up. She believed she was on something to strengthen her heart; perhaps Digoxin I thought. Could I be sure? What dose might she be taking?

I had no idea without her records. Fortunately, she lived only a few streets away and this tolerant grandmother agreed to go home and return with her remaining tablets and packaging.

Eventually, the last of over twenty patients entered, a mother holding a little boy firmly by the hand. He was suffering from a painful ear. I searched in the desk's drawers for an auroscope and found a rather old-fashioned model and a half full bottle of Irish whiskey. The device was dead but the boy was very much alive and racing around the room ignoring his mother's ineffectual commands to sit still. Clearly, he was not terribly unwell. A further search through the drawers found some hidden batteries. Now armed with an auroscope which produced a bright light. I attempted to examine the child's ear. Not only was this a bit of a struggle but the defective instrument refused to focus on the eardrum. Some component was undoubtedly missing. I wrote out a script for an antibiotic to be brought to the local pharmacy and for some soothing anti-inflammatory ear drops . The mother was happy that these had worked once before. I advised them to return on Monday if the medicine proved ineffective.

It was well after 7.30 p.m. when the old lady reappeared. I was waiting with the caretaker who was not amused at the delay. I was able to provide her with the prescription she needed, and she was embarrassingly effusive in her thanks. She was of an age to have appreciated the introduction of the National Health Service and the advent of free treatment for all. This attitude from someone who clearly lived on a limited income reinforced my strong belief in the NHS, even if this particular surgery was perhaps not the best it had to offer.

Learning in this way about the demands and delivery of health care outside the safety and efficiency of a major teaching hospital, was a chastening experience for someone still relatively naive and altruistic.

I felt it was unlikely that I would accept another offer to work in such circumstances. I discussed the encounter with my hospital colleague and my concerns about the apparently chaotic way in which the surgery seemed to operate. He suggested it provided an important locally available service and probably functioned much more efficiently with someone who knew the clientele individually. We agreed that he would take up the issue with the central Practice as to how appropriate it was to engage inexperienced locum doctors to work there. On reflection, keeping this outlying clinic functioning probably saved old ladies and others from travelling considerable distances through potentially dangerous streets.

The Royal College of Physicians

Our wedding was set for the week after Anne took her final nursing examinations. This just gave us just over a year to accumulate some capital, which I planned to deposit in a building society account, with a view to obtaining a mortgage. I hoped extra finance might be earned from further GP locum work. However, in order to advance my paediatric career, I also needed to gain some postgraduate qualifications.

The path to more senior posts depended on becoming a member of the Royal College of Physicians. The qualification was an essential ticket to a consultant position. This entailed undertaking a two-part examination. If passed, this conferred the privilege of writing the letters MRCP after one's name. The first part was a written test of medical knowledge and theory. Questions covered the entire spectrum of human disease. Some of my peers had already overcome this hurdle, despite an apparent pass rate among candidates of only 20%. So, I spent long evenings and weekends consuming Cecil and Loeb's *Textbook of Internal Medicine*, alongside large volumes of coffee and many, many packets of digestive biscuits. After six months of burning the midnight oil, I undertook the examination - but was gutted when I received a letter informing me that I had not reached the required standard. This was the first examination I had ever failed. In the past, I had even managed to overcome a mental block for foreign languages to pass a GCSE (General Certificate of Secondary Education) in French, admittedly by a narrow margin. All I had to show for my recent hard work was an extra three or four kg in weight.

Somewhat depressed, I sought advice from my professor, feeling guilty that I had not fulfilled his expectations when he appointed me as a junior tutor in his department. He treated me with the kindly attitude he usually reserved for his young patients.

"The first part of the MRCP is a completely adult illness-oriented assessment," he declared, "and think about it, since you qualified, nearly all your experience has been in paediatrics. You have only spent three months in adult neurology. I think you'll agree you have no postgraduate experience in general medicine. I've found that my trainees in paediatrics often have trouble with the part one."

He looked thoughtful for a minute.

"Based on your experience, maybe you should take the Diploma in Child Health instead? It's not as tough… Then you should go and get some more experience on an adult ward before you try again. A move to an adult medicine post for six months to gain more general experience should do it. If you are successful, as I expect, move back to paediatrics and by then you will be able to opt to undertake the clinical second part of the MRCP in Paediatric Medicine".

It was wise advice. I found the Child Health Diploma paper straightforward, and I was able to successfully diagnose each child presented to me in the practical clinical examination, which was held in Dublin. I clearly remember the first patient I was shown, who had the typical rash of measles and pneumonia, rarely seen today despite Dr Andrew Wakefield's malign influence on vaccination rates, caused by a subsequently discredited research study suggesting a link between the Measles, Mumps, and Rubella

Vaccine (MMR) and autism. I can recall not just the miserable child but also the unique name on the door of the isolation room. It required two plastic strips to contain the title: "The Blessed Guardian Angel of St. Patrick Ward".

When my interrogation was finished, I mentally thanked the guardian angel for apparently also watching over me. It was much later that I learned the angel's name was Victor and his task was to assist Patrick in this life's mission of bringing Christianity to Ireland. Perhaps he had taken me, a sceptic, under his wings, too.

A return to adult medicine

Back on track, I was seconded to the adult academic medical unit, in which I had spent several attachments as an undergraduate. Compared to my previous posts, the out-of-hours work was comparatively light. The greatest demands were from the weekly "take in" days and weekends, when we accepted all emergency admissions for the entire city. On a busy winter's night, we might admit 20 or more patients, although we never had 20 empty beds in our own ward at the start of the day. These men and women had a wide spectrum of conditions: heart failure, stroke, diabetes, gastric ulcers, inflammatory bowel disease, bronchitis, pneumonia, asthma. They were rarely young. Some had more than one diagnosis and were perhaps alcoholic or showing signs of dementia. Following a provisional diagnosis in the A&E department, they'd arrive in our ward, where we would record the clinical findings in detail and initiate treatment. As part of this workup, we would order and interpret a range of investigations for presentation next morning. Armed with the results, I would join the mammoth ward round, led by one of the professors of medicine. The supporting cast generally included lowly house physicians, registrars, the senior ward sister, and several medical students. There were two aims. Firstly, to confirm that each diagnosis and prescribed treatment plan was correct; and secondly, to review every patient before the start of the afternoon outpatient clinics at 2 p.m.. (I was allocated to clinics in Rheumatology and General Medicine.) These ward rounds were physically exhausting and intellectually challenging after being awake all night. As planned, I was studying and learning in depth about the whole range of adult disease.

We attempted in various ways to lighten the intensity of these "grand rounds". For instance, we discreetly awarded a weekly gold medal for the biggest faux pas during the patient presentations and teaching, which were an integral part of the morning. Special delight was taken in awarding this to a high-flying senior registrar, who had confused two similar medical terms or conditions as he expounded knowledgeably to the impressionable students. The medal was created from a metal intravenous bottle top and a gold ribbon from a gifted box of chocolates. We all recognised such a minor error was merely a slip of the tongue on his part- but in an exhausted state, with serious illness and responsibility all around us, any humour was a welcome relief.

Our highly efficient senior sister had a distinctive red uniform and a wicked underlying sense of humour. The Professor decreed that cigarette smoking should be banned in his unit, well in advance of any hospital policy. She was tasked with implementing his edict, despite packets of cigarettes being readily available at the hospital shop.

A week or so later, as we progressed down the female ward, the professor stopped, held up his hand and with a look of disbelief asked, "Sister, can I smell tobacco smoke?"

Smiling coyly, she apologetically confirmed his suspicion.

"Have we not banned cigarettes from the ward?" he demanded.

"Oh yes sir," she replied and pulled back the curtain from around the next bed, in which sat a wrinkled little old lady, "but dear Agnes here always likes her clay pipe of tobacco with her morning cup of tea."

Agnes smiled benignly at the eminent doctor; a traditional Irish white clay pipe clamped between her gums.

"Do you want me to include pipes in the ban too?" sister asked with false innocence. The Prof closed his eyes, shook his head slightly and said firmly, "I do."

He then turned back to the patient we had just been discussing, allowing himself a wry smile, permitting us all to have a brief laugh to acknowledge that he knew he had been set up, rather than disobeyed.

Halfway through the morning, sister usually vanished, and was replaced by the second in command - a blue-uniformed junior sister or a staff nurse. As we reached the end of the first of our two main wards, the welcome smell of percolating coffee would drift in from the tutorial room. Sister would hold court there, as the professor tested us on some obscure clinical point

"What do you think the salt content of a pint of Guinness stout is?" he once asked, suggesting it might have relevance as to why a patient, a Mr McCrory, developed heart failure after drinking 10 pints on the evening of his admission to hospital. When no one came up with a definite answer, he picked on a medical student.

"Miss McCord, can you find this out and educate us all on next time we meet?"

A few days later we reached Mr McCrory's bed again, only to find it empty. Assuming he was at the bathroom, we moved on. Shortly, one of the hospital security staff approached. He drew sister aside.

"It's your patient Mr McCrory" he said quietly. "He is on the bus outside the hospital and refusing to get off for the driver, or for us"

Someone asked if he had signed himself out against medical advice. He had not.

"Actually, the real problem is that he is completely naked, apart from his hospital armband," the security guard explained, "and he has been approaching other people who board, trying to borrow the fare. I'm afraid there are a couple of elderly ladies who fled from the bus and are in quite a distressed state in the front gate lodge."

Sister grabbed a dressing gown and commandeered the house physician.

The three rushed off and a few minutes later they reappeared with the elderly patient, now wrapped in the hospital issue dressing gown. One arm was held gently by sister and the other more firmly by the houseman.

" I was only nipping out for a pint." he protested.

My adventurous tightrope walker patients, who became escapees from the Children's ward, had only wanted to go home, but had been more successful than Mr McCrory in reaching a pub.

I don't think we ever learnt the salt content of Guinness.

Hello again

Over my six months, I encountered a man who was repeatedly admitted to us from the Accident and Emergency department with chest pains and a suspected coronary heart attack. On each occasion, no evidence of this was found, and he returned home reassured. On a more detailed review of his medical history, we eventually learned that the emergency cardiac ambulance had rushed to his home several times in the past, at the request of doctors from the General Practitioner service. He had several brief admissions to the coronary care unit as a result. After exhaustive investigations, the cardiology team explained to him that he had no evidence of any heart disease. He was advised this specialist ambulance would not attend for him again. Now he was turning up of his own volition at the hospital A&E. Once more, we explained that with repeated normal assessments by two teams it was unlikely he would need to be admitted again, as we were certain his heart was normal and strong. He was horrified and offended at a suggestion that he might like to discuss his fears with a psychiatrist, and refused the offer.

We didn't see him for months. We worried that perhaps he had cried wolf once too often. Our ward clerk, who scoured the death notices daily in the local papers, assured us his name had not appeared. One day, towards the end of my time, I entered the elevator on my way to an outpatient clinic and there he was, smartly dressed and wearing dark glasses. I asked how he was keeping. Despite the shades, he seemed to recognise me and informed me his angina had settled. He volunteered that he was on his way to see his ophthalmologist.

"Yes, I noticed the sunglasses. What has been the problem?" I asked, almost immediately regretting the question.

"I'm progressively losing my eyesight," he said, sadly. "Worst of all, the eye specialists haven't been able to work out why."

Before I could speak, the elevator stopped and, as the doors opened, he flicked out a collapsible white stick, and tapped his way out.

Later in my career I thought of him when I encountered or considered a diagnosis of Munchausen Disease by Proxy, a condition where a parent gains medical attention by exaggerating or claiming fake symptoms in a child, or even by causing real symptoms. In one instance I encountered, this was achieved by regularly and surreptitiously adding little restaurant sachets of salt to an infant's bottled milk, which was otherwise prepared and supplied by the hospital. (Baron Von Munchausen was a semi fictional eighteenth-century German nobleman infamous for his outrageous tall tales of his adventures).

After six months, it was time to resit the first part of the Royal College examination. My additional experience, the extra time available for study (and sleep) and the structured formal teaching sessions in adult medicine would hopefully benefit me. One unforgettable, demanding section of the assessment was sitting, with perhaps one hundred other candidates, staring at slides projected onto a large screen in a lecture theatre. A new slide, of perhaps, an x-ray, a set of blood testresults, or a picture of a patient, appeared every two minutes, before which a diagnosis had to be written on an answer sheet.The sensation that others were already writing as I stared at the slide, was panic inducing.

Despite the pressure, when the results were published, I'd been successful. It was time to return to my first love.

6. Working to rule

In 2016, a junior doctors' strike in the UK made headlines as the unpopular Minister of Health, Jeremy Hunt, sought, and eventually managed to impose a new contract on them. The dispute was reminiscent of my experience 40 years before when, again, junior doctors were demoralised by long hours, with frequent nights and weekends on call with very little or no sleep. Rarely, in the arguments around the 1974/75 dispute, was there any discussion about the competing demands of work and family life for young doctors. In paediatrics, we were trying to balance the need to care for both our own and other people's children. The concept of work/life balance was not part of the language of the day. It was, however, of great importance to Anne and me, as our firstborn arrived around that time. Many of us were working these long hours while bringing up young families. Perhaps returning to the warmth of home and children helped keep us sane and enabled us to cope. The birth of our little boy and, in time, his two sisters again made real the ancient phrase, "The gift of a child".

Young doctors on the frontline recognised that working to the limits of exhaustion posed a risk to their patients. I can remember, for instance, once falling asleep while talking to a staff nurse on the phone in the middle of the night. A colleague, who was best man at our wedding, out for a meal after a long shift, fell asleep in the restaurant toilet and missed the dessert course.

At the heart of our grievances, even then, were understaffing and the lack of remuneration for the excessive hours we worked. A potential breakthrough in negotiations between the British Medical Association and the Government came in 1975, when there was an agreement that the junior's salary would in future be for a basic 40-hour week.

Subsequently, however, Barbara Castle, the Minister of Health, cunningly announced that her calculated hourly rate would be based on the current wage divided by the average number of hours worked by the junior doctors. This meant some doctors would actually be paid even less than before.

The BMA decided to call a strike in response to what they considered an underhand action, in order to obtain a more reasonable settlement. Mrs. Castle was determined to show just how tough a politician she was by facing down her opponents. She had assessed that the doctors would inevitably crack and, as professionals, put their patients first. A victory, she hoped, would mark her out as a potential future leader of her party, if not the country. The doctors did not strike but instead began a Work to Rule, only showing up for the 40 hours a week of the initial agreement.

In paediatrics, we decided that even this action was morally unacceptable when looking after ill children, as there were unlikely to be adequate numbers of consultant staff to take over, cover gaps and ensure the patients' safety 24 hours a day, seven days a week. I strongly supported this stance.

In the event, the minister capitulated, agreeing a contract enshrining the basic, fully paid 40-hour week, with an extra 30% payment rate for hours worked beyond this There was also to be full-rate payment for extra hours worked to fill gaps in a rota. The extra hours payment rate was at only one third of the daytime rate, unlike overtime payment to other workers in industry. Nevertheless, for those working 120 hours per week their income increased by 60%.

The problem of staff fatigue and risk to patient safety remained unsolved, however, and was still a bone of contention in 2016.

In 1974, there was another industrial action which affected the whole community: The Ulster Workers Strike. It was organised by people opposed to the agreement made at Sunningdale to set up a Northern Ireland power-sharing executive at Stormont, composed of representatives from a broad spectrum of political parties. It was hoped that this arrangement might bring peace. This strike lasted for two weeks. The mainly protestant workforce in the power supply industry succeeded in significantly reducing electricity output resulting in power cuts. Many roads were blocked encouraging workers to stay at home, although the main roads generally remained open. I found, when I attempted to drive to the hospital one morning, that I was stopped at a roadblock, set up by the paramilitary Ulster Defence Association. I refused to return home, and was subjected to some verbal abuse. Eventually, I was able to persuade the young men manning the makeshift barricade that doctors might be needed in hospitals if events got nasty, especially if any of them needed treatment. I was waved through, having omitted to mention I was going to the children's department rather than A&E.

The Power-sharing Executive soon collapsed.

The final hurdle

Shortly after settling back into paediatrics, I was invited to attend part two of the MRCP clinical examinations in London. Before the date indicated in the instructions, I discovered that one of my nursing colleagues had worked for some time in the hospital at which I was to present myself. As she reminisced about her time there, she related that the spectrum of disease differed somewhat from that in our local population, partly because of the numbers of children from Afro-Caribbean families. She advised me that I should swot up on conditions like sickle cell disease. I had never encountered this inherited condition, in which affected individuals become anaemic due to an abnormal form of haemoglobin, the oxygen-carrying molecule in red blood cells. This causes the flexible, round cells to deform into a sickle or crescent shape, with the potential to block blood vessels. It is most likely to be found in people originating in tropical Africa or the Middle East. I took her advice and revised this - and other related topics - in my hotel room on the evening of a restless night prior to the examination. Next morning, I boarded the underground train for Clapham North, near the examination venue, the Belgrave Children's Hospital.

As I left the station, concentrating on remembering the directions I had been given, I was somewhat taken aback to be approached by an attractive young woman, dressed in red, who asked me, "Would you like some more?"

I stuttered a negative reply, but she pressed a narrow red carton into my hand and moved on to intercept the next passenger. I stared at the free promotional packet of extra-long "More" cigarettes, then hastened on, all thoughts of tropical disease now gone. A few minutes later, checking in with the examinations officer in an old Victorian red brick building, I realised I was still carrying the packet of cigarettes and quickly stuffed them into my pocket to avoid creating a poor impression.

For what was called the "long case", I was introduced to a pleasant black child and his mother and left for an hour to obtain a history, perform an examination and form a diagnosis. It was immediately obvious that the little boy had a severe neurological disability, possibly cerebral palsy. Despite his problems, he was a happy child and his mother was friendly and keen to give me all the information I needed. He was born healthy but had been in hospital many times for blood transfusions. His worst illness was when he developed meningitis. She confirmed my suspicion that he had sickle cell disease and helped me construct a family tree of affected individuals. Concluding that she was very knowledgeable, I inquired about her occupation and learnt she was a nursing assistant in the hospital. I knew from my reading that children with this condition were susceptible to certain bacterial infections and she recognised the name of the specific organism I suggested. Her son was very ticklish and enjoyed being examined. By the time my interrogator arrived, I had all the facts marshalled to accurately present the case. I thanked both the boy and his mum for their help and proceeded to be taken to make spot diagnoses on a number of "minor cases" without much difficulty.

The final hurdle was an oral discussion, or viva. This went reasonably well until the last few minutes.

"What diseases would you say are more common in Irish children than in children here on the mainland?" asked the Professor. I made some suggestions relating to the incidence of coeliac disease, spina bifida, and cystic fibrosis, before running out of ideas.

"What about juvenile schizophrenia?" he asked.

I admitted I had never seen a child with this condition.

"Surely you must have," he retorted, in what I considered a rather condescending way.

"Given the high incidence of alcoholism in the Irish, and increased risk of the condition in the children of alcoholics, it must also be higher."

His attitude triggered a response, offered without forethought. I suggested his caricature of Irish fathers was possibly inaccurate and that I was not aware of any sound statistical evidence that there were more alcoholics per head of the population in Ireland than in England or Scotland.

Silence fell. He looked at me for a few seconds until, fortunately, a buzzer sounded.

"Thank you, doctor, it seems our time is up," he said, proffering a hand, which I shook.

Retracing my footsteps to the tube station, I reflected that I had probably blown my chances. I could hear my mother saying, "Son, sometimes you need to hold your tongue."

In 2021, WHO reported an identical incidence of alcoholism in Ireland and the UK.

When, in due course, a letter arrived with the Royal College crest on the envelope, I opened it in trepidation.

"I am pleased to inform you…"

7. Moonlighting, night calls

The violence in Northern Ireland reached a peak in the mid-1970s, resulting in several hundred deaths each year. The British Army and the Royal Ulster Constabulary patrolled the streets of Belfast and security roadblocks were commonplace. Anyone travelling at night was very likely to be stopped, their identity checked, their person and car searched. In some areas, roadblocks might be manned by paramilitary groups or vigilantes. Not surprisingly, some family doctors were reluctant to provide an out of hours domiciliary service in those difficult days. A local medical practitioner recognised a potential market and set up a commercial Night Doctor Bureau to address the problem. GPs could subcontract their night calls to the bureau, which would employ junior doctors willing to respond to calls. I worked an occasional evening for the bureau for a short time, ignoring, a little naively in retrospect, the potential risks. In day-to-day life, like most of the population, I had become acclimatised to the security situation. Newly married, with a mortgage to pay and a home to furnish, the remuneration was attractive. I no longer needed to spend my free evenings in study, having obtained the higher qualifications which were the gateway to consultant training.

All sides in the conflict - government forces, republican and loyalist groups - were aware of the role the night bureau doctors played in serving the whole community, irrespective of political persuasion or religion. Our cars displayed large signs attached to the folded down sun visor on the passenger side, stating, "DOCTOR ON CALL". Generally, this conferred immunity from harm. Often the evening switchboard operator at the bureau was, by day, employed in the children's hospital and, when I worked a shift, she selectively referred any calls involving children to me.

Punctured

On one occasion, I was on my way to see someone with an acute asthma attack when an irregular bump from a rear wheel indicated that I had a puncture. The roads in the area were often littered with broken glass, possibly debris from milk bottle petrol bombs, following confrontations between opposing factions. Cursing my luck, I pulled over and got out to change the wheel.

I was in a solidly republican area of Belfast. To confuse British army patrols, and delay their efforts should they carry out a raid to arrest a suspect, street names were often painted out or replaced by alternative, Irish language versions. Here, presumably for the same reason, the streetlights had also been damaged or turned off. In the darkness, I opened the car boot and, feeling rather vulnerable, shivered in the cold night air. To my horror, I realised the spare tyre was also flat. This was in the pre-mobile phone era, but I had a two-way radio with which I could contact the office. As I returned to the front seat to find it, two shadowy figures in dark clothes appeared and, looking me over, asked, "Do you have a problem?"

Another person hung back at the street corner. I quickly told them who I was, and about the flat tyres. They walked around the car suspiciously, then one asked me where exactly I was going. I explained and gave the name and address of the patient, which was nearby.

"Right Doc," said the older of the two, "give us your keys". A command rather than a request.

I momentarily hesitated, thinking this would be the last I would see of my car and wondering what might happen to me.

"You do your house call and we'll sort out the punctures. Don't rush yourself."

I had no alternative. I retrieved my medical bag and slipped the radio into it, hoping they didn't notice. I set off up the hill, turned left and found the house I was planning to visit. The patient was wheezing quite badly, so I administered a slow intravenous dose of a bronchodilating drug, with good effect. As I counted out a starter dose of antibiotic tablets, known by the trade name Penbritin, I mentioned the fate of my car to the family, and sat down to write a prescription. As the man's breathing settled, a delaying cup of tea was suggested. As this was prepared, I explained I needed to radio the office to explain I might not be able to take further calls. I stepped into the hallway and reported my predicament. Eventually, leaving the house after a judicious delay, I was accompanied down the short front garden to the street by the lady of the house. Amazingly, outside sat my car, the rear tyre fully inflated and the keys in the ignition. Both of us were delighted, my new friend perhaps not quite as surprised as me. I was also extremely grateful, but there was no one around to thank. I asked the lady to convey my gratitude to the local paramilitary unit, if she knew who to speak to.

"I'll see what I can do," she said, "but it was probably just the lads from the black taxi depot. Thanks for coming… and safe home."

Later, I found the spare tyre had also been repaired.

A security raid

A friend was not quite so lucky. He was visiting a home in another part of the city late in the evening when the front door crashed open and an army snatch squad filled the house. The three occupants were quickly rounded up and roughly marched out to an armoured personnel carrier (known locally as a Pig, due to its ugly squat appearance). Phillip was taken too, despite protesting loudly that he was a doctor. The squaddies were not interested, being under orders to arrest all the male adults in the house - and also, it seemed, those in adjacent ones. The street was sealed off by army vehicles, police, and troops, who held protesting local residents back while the raid was rapidly carried out. In the background, women created an intimidating cacophony by beating dustbin lids with sticks, alerting the whole area to what was happening.

In 15 minutes, the exercise was over, and Phillip found himself being held in a nearby police station. He demanded to see an officer and after some time was interviewed by a supercilious type, who pointed out that the doctor paraphernalia could be just "a bloody good disguise". After what seemed like hours, he was informed that the Night Doctor Bureau had vouched for him and he was free to go. Perhaps the security forces had found the individual they were searching for. He never found out any details, the event wasn't reported in the media and, of course, he never received any apology. He had yet another risky experience to endure - being taken in an armoured police Land Rover, back through an area where the Royal Ulster Constabulary was less than popular, to complete the house call and retrieve his car.

Most call outs were routine and today would not warrant a night visit. The unique local circumstances mitigated against unnecessary trips to Accident and Emergency by those with minor complaints. This reluctance even applied to some who were seriously in need of attention. Conversely, there was less hesitation by some in calling out the family doctor.

An obstetric dilemma

One evening, I had a request by radio to visit a pregnant woman who thought she might be in labour, although she was not due for a few weeks. I pointed out that such calls could only be undertaken by someone who had the appropriate qualification. Shortly afterwards, the switchboard operator came back to me saying there was no appropriate doctor on the rota for that evening. I advised her that the responsibility then lay with the patient's own doctor. I learned that he could not be contacted. As it was near the end of my shift, the operator, now desperate, pleaded with me at least to call in on the young lady. She pointed out that I would pass near the address on my way home. I was assured she would continue to attempt to reach the GP, so reluctantly, I agreed to perform the visit rather than leave the patient unattended, mainly to salve my conscience.

I detoured as requested and was soon driving down the street, which was a mile or so from my childhood home. The house was easily identified as the one in which every light blazed out. My knock at the door was answered instantaneously. I was shown into the main living room where the expectant mother was lying on the sofa. A contraction gripped her as I stepped through the door but it was her face that drew my attention. I recognised a girl who had been a near neighbour and classmate when I was in primary school. She had lived only a few houses from my family and our mothers were good friends. Twenty or so years earlier, my brothers and I played regularly with her and her sisters and we were in each other's houses almost daily. As an expectant mother, she was so glad to see me that she didn't even consider any embarrassment I might have in examining her. I restricted myself to palpating her abdomen and was quickly convinced she was well established in labour. I checked there was an audible regular foetal heartbeat with my stethoscope, while thinking quickly about what to do. I had not delivered a baby since I was a medical student several years before.

113

I was faced with someone in her first pregnancy, experiencing a situation in which I should never have become involved.

I told her she did not have long to go before the baby was born and explained I had only called by until a more experienced doctor could get there. I reassured her that I could deliver the baby if need be, but did not wish to embarrass her by performing an internal examination myself, unless it became necessary. I stepped out of the room to call the bureau on the radio. The response was worrying. They still had no one available with obstetric credentials. The contractions were now more frequent. I decided to call an ambulance and get my childhood friend to the safety of the maternity hospital.

Picking up the house phone, I called the neonatal unit where I worked and was well known.

"I need a favour," I explained rapidly to the nurse in charge. "Can you tell me who is on the flying squad tonight? I've run into an emergency and need their help. I don't have time to go into all the details." I heard a rustling of paper and then she named a colleague who was a good friend. She had detected the worry in my voice.

"Can you get hold of him and impress on him that I am anxious to speak to him at once? Please give him this number, there's little time to lose."

Shortly, he came through on the house phone. I told him I was in a bit of a panic and explained the situation with the lack of obstetric cover.

"The problem is the flying squad is for life or death emergencies, serious haemorrhages and that sort of thing," he said uncertainly. "This is just a girl in labour. It happens every day of the week. I'm sure you'll be able to cope. Why don't you just get an ordinary ambulance?"

"Gary, I have a bad feeling about this. I'm afraid something will go wrong and this girl is an old friend from way back. Our parents are friends. I'm caught in an awkward situation. When we were young, I used to call her mum my auntie. Please do me a favour and come? Now!"

"Well, if it was anyone else but you," came the response. He was a generous sort of bloke and recognised my predicament and anxiety.

114

"Just pray we don't get another emergency call. I'll get the team on board and we'll be on our way in a couple of minutes."

After giving him the name and address details, I returned to sit with the patient, checking her blood pressure, monitoring the frequency and strength of her contractions and reassuring her. I told her and her husband that I had sent for the maternity hospital's flying squad - only because I didn't usually deliver babies myself but rather took care of them after they were born. Chatting about our school days, I did the best I could to appear calm and communicate that I was merely making sure everything would go perfectly for her and the baby. They knew I had listened to its heart beat several times and it was fine.

In a very short time, Gary was there with a midwife and two ambulance men. I discreetly retired with the husband to the kitchen, where he had been preparing a cup of tea. Soon, my old school friend, expertly assessed, was on a stretcher trolley and heading out the door to the ambulance, with the midwife in control. I managed to say a quick "thank you" to my colleague, who was anxious to get back to base quickly, but informed me quietly he was fairly sure they would get there in plenty of time. As the ambulance pulled away, I breathed a sigh of relief, swearing to myself that doing this sort of favour was a mistake I would never make again.

At home, I fell into a restless sleep after the tension of the evening's final events. An hour or two later the phone rang. It was Gary.

"We were bloody fortunate to get your friend into the labour ward on time. Fifteen minutes after we arrived, she delivered a five-pound healthy baby boy. But you'll not believe what happened next!"

He had my full attention. I listened with trepidation.

"I was about to give her the usual injection to contract the uterus down but first did the standard post-delivery check examination. To my surprise, I discovered there was another wee one in there; undiagnosed twins! Only the parents were more shocked than me!

"It gave me quite a fright, thinking of what might have happened if I hadn't examined her again. Obviously, her own doctor hadn't recognised the twin pregnancy. The second delivery was a bit more difficult than the first, but they are all well".

I think I just said, "Shit!" or some similar expletive, before thanking him (and God) profusely, no longer feeling guilty about having broken the normal rules by calling him out.

Foetal ultrasound scanning prevents such dramas today.

A month later, I happened to be washing my car outside my parent's house where we were visiting, when a Ford Cortina pulled up and I heard a woman call out my name. The passenger door swung open and the twins' grandmother, who I had not seen for years, climbed out. She rushed over to me.

"Thank you for everything you did that night for my girl and the babies," she gushed.

"You were absolutely brilliant, and so calm handling everything, when you discovered she was having twins."

She threw her arms around me and I was subjected to an enormous hug. Smiling, she stepped back.

"That GP of ours had missed the twins completely, even though he saw her regularly. But you made the diagnosis immediately you laid a hand on her tummy. I heard how you were on the phone for the flying squad within seconds. Thank God it was you who arrived instead of him."

She went on for several minutes, as I tried to interrupt with the truth.

"Twins can be difficult to diagnose." I protested. "And it was actually the flying squad doctor who spotted the twins when they got to hospital."

She refused to be deterred from her belief, casting me in the role of some sort of hero. She smiled knowingly at me, inclined her head, and tapped her nose with her forefinger,

"I know what you doctors are like, always covering for each other. You can't fool your old auntie."

The last night call

My final house visit on behalf of the bureau had a very different ending. After treating an elderly man with a urinary infection, I checked back to base and the switchboard gave me two calls. One was designated urgent - a man with chest pains. The second was a woman with a possible respiratory infection. I went immediately to see the patient with the potential coronary thrombosis. The chest discomfort from which he was suffering seemed to be indigestion, precipitated by drinking several pints of beer following a greasy meal of fish and chips. The symptoms improved quickly with a couple of antacid tablets.

I then drove to a run-down area in the east of the city, already designated for redevelopment, and parked outside an old three-story terrace. There was no response to knocking on the door, from which paint was flaking. I knocked again, much harder this time, and the door creaked and moved inwards a little. I pushed it open and entered a rather musty smelling, unlit hallway. I could hear the noise of a television from behind the door at the end of the dark passageway. I knocked on it and tentatively turned the handle. Again, there was no light in the room, but in the glow of the television screen sat a man watching a show with two small children.

"Hello," I spoke into the gloom. "I'm the Doctor. Was it you who called about someone with a bad chest?"

He stood up, indicating a couch against the back wall, and said, "It's my wife. She has a lot of trouble with her chest and her breathing has been getting worse this evening. I think she has the Flu. She has just lain down for a rest."

I walked over to the young woman, repeating to her that I was the doctor. She did not reply and, assuming she was asleep, I knelt down to wake her. As I touched her shoulder, her arm and hand fell down limply over the side of the sofa. Shocked, I instinctively checked for her pulse with my own heart pounding. I couldn't locate it. Although warm, her limbs lacked any tone. A feeling of panic began to grip me. I turned to the husband, suppressing a niggle of anger, who was paying little attention to us as he held the little ones. I called loudly over the sound of the TV, asking him to turn the light on, quickly. I told him I was worried about his wife and examining her was difficult in the dark.

I was pulling open her clothes and still getting no response as I made my demand. With unsteady hands, I got my stethoscope out and set the diaphragm on her chest.

There was no heartbeat.

In the distance, I heard her husband apologising that the light bulb had gone. He opened a door into a small kitchen off the main room. Light from

117

there flooded across the room. I could see my patient's lips were blue. She did not appear to be breathing. I stepped quickly over to the man. I spoke quietly but forcefully.

"Your wife is desperately ill, please move the children out of here and up to bed."

He wasn't convinced. "They will be all right here, just you go ahead."

I grabbed his arm and quickly pulled him a couple of steps into the kitchen.

'I'm desperately sorry to be blunt," I said to him rapidly. "I'm afraid their mum is terribly ill and may have passed away, or is close to it. You need to get the children out of the room. I need to start heart massage and try to revive her."

He was immediately distraught and rushed to her.

"This can't be happening. I made her a cup of tea only twenty minutes ago" he cried. Indeed, there was a cup, half-full of tepid tea, on the floor beside her.

The next hours passed in a blur of frantic activity. My resuscitation attempts were performed on automatic pilot, programmed from past experience. I called in on the radio for the emergency services. My memory is vague, but all my efforts were in vain, as were those of the ambulance crew I summoned. The bureau was able to contact the family doctor, and informed me he was on his way. Relatives arrived and the children were spirited away. Neighbours came to help their father, who was beyond grief. I tried to reassure him that he had done all he could. I emphasised to him that he could not have foreseen that his wife's heart could give out with the influenza at her age. The words arrhythmia and cardiac arrest probably did not register. It was a relief to hand over to the general practitioner, who knew the family, and the woman's past history of chest problems, well. He had the difficult task of explaining that a postmortem might be required. By law, any sudden death is required to be reported to the coroner. The duty police became involved and, as tactfully as possible, collected preliminary statements. This was even more distressing for the family. For them, these were life-changing events, never to be forgotten. It had been a tragic night. I decided within days that I had finished with the night bureau.

118

Later, I would reflect that these experiences at the front line of family medicine gave me a valuable perspective. Those of us who practiced only in the hospital environment, ran the danger of almost living in another world from our patients. Somehow, we needed to get nearer to, or at least understand, how and where they spent their daily lives.

8. A teenage pregnancy

A call from the labour ward alerted me that an emergency Caesarean Section was underway. A paediatrician was needed immediately. I had just commenced my first post as a registrar, the promotion gained as a result of becoming a member of the Royal College. I arrived breathless at the unfamiliar operating theatre, hastily pulled on a sterile gown, a hat, clean surgical boots and scrubbed up. I was just in time to receive the baby from the obstetrician's hands. The infant cried weakly.

We placed him under an overhead heater and, as a midwife gently dried off the amniotic fluid from his body, I checked his breathing and rapid heartbeat with my small neonatal stethoscope. The nurse efficiently and gently cleared fluid from the nose and throat using a simple oral suction device. This consisted of a short length of soft tubing and a fluid trap that prevented anything being aspirated into her mouth. The baby protested vigorously and loudly at this assault. I was relieved and delighted to hear his noisy objections.

"Weight four pounds 12 ounces," said the midwife shortly. "A little on the small side, but so is the mother."

The immediate crisis was over.

We transported the baby a short distance to the Special Care Baby Unit (SCBU), safe and warm in a portable incubator. Later my new chief, a woman of long experience, joined me for our routine daily round, during which she performed or supervised a meticulous examination of every child in each of the wards, finishing with the babies in the neonatal unit. Finally, we sat down to review our decisions over a cup of tea. She was especially interested in the details of the baby who had needed to be delivered by caesarean earlier. I explained that this was judged necessary because of signs of foetal distress during a premature labour, with a dipping foetal heart rate developing with each contraction, and because the mother was becoming exhausted. She had gone into labour unexpectedly at 35 weeks in a nearby nursing home. This establishment, I understood, was run by a religious order. I learnt with surprise from the SCBU Sister that the mother was still a schoolgirl and did not live locally but had a home address many miles away in a rural area. She knew more detail of the background story and revealed that the girl had not been booked for delivery in our hospital. Having finished the recap, and our tea, my wily boss spoke to me.

"We have one patient whom we have yet to see, doctor."

I reassured her that we have not missed any of the babies, but she looked directly at me over the top of her spectacles.

"There is a child in the maternity ward. Not only do we need to see her, but we need to be sure our colleagues in social services are aware of today's events. That child will need support and protection. She, too, is our responsibility for now. The senior social worker may involve the police, depending on the mother's age and the identity of the father."

I think I heard her mutter, "There must be no cover up," as she climbed the stairs ahead of me.

I looked at the sister, who pursed her lips and nodded grimly. I followed the doctor's determined footsteps. Her prim demeanour concealed a sharp and astute intelligence.

Over the months I was to learn a lot from this formidable woman, and even if sometimes her approach was a little unconventional, it was always thorough.

Puzzling seizures

A girl was brought to the hospital on several occasions after apparently having a seizure at home. Each time, she appeared to make a complete recovery, with no residual signs of harm detected in the emergency department. When she attended yet again, her parents repeated the perplexing story of brief unexplained turns without residual clinical signs or ill effects. A paediatric opinion was requested. The child seemed fine when examined, but I decided that since the episodes, although brief, were recurrent, she should be admitted for observation, further investigations and discussion. A few days later, on our rounds, the nursing staff reported observing two jerking episodes, both when her mother was present. They told us the fits were not typical of others they had observed, and tentatively ventured the opinion that they might be contrived. I reported that her blood analyses, including sugar levels and metabolic studies, were normal, as was an electroencephalogram brain wave pattern. My consultant performed a full neurological examination again and, like me, found nothing of note. Some minutes later, as we assessed a little boy with pneumonia at the other side of the six-bedded bay, there was quite a disturbance as the girl writhed and jerked on her bed.

"Dear, Oh, dear!" exclaimed my senior medical colleague loudly. "Dorothy is having one of her turns. Quickly nurse, fix her nightie, all the boys can see her pants!"

The dramatic movements ceased immediately as the little girl, blushing, frantically pulled down her night dress. The curtains were drawn around her bed and we were waved away as my mentor gently sat down on it, to have a sympathetic chat with the child. Later, a more delicate discussion took place with her mother and father. It transpired that they were in the middle of divorce proceedings but were doing all they could to minimise the effect on their children. Their daughter, for her part, it seemed, was doing all she could to hold on to the two most important people in her life.

Burn's night

It was unusual to call a consultant into the hospital at night. Not that they were unwilling to come and help or advise, if asked. It was almost a matter of pride for a registrar to be able to cope with almost any problem. Often, this was with input and assistance from skilled and experienced nursing colleagues. Night staff, especially, were likely to have been nursing ill children for decades and to have seen almost every possible scenario. There was a certain satisfaction in being able to identify a problem, by phone, to the consultant on call, and explain how it had been successfully resolved. By the time I became a young consultant, I sometimes found I could not return to sleep after similar calls and ended up driving to the hospital - if only to confirm that, indeed, I was not needed. As a registrar, the most testing and unforgettable problems seemed inevitably to present outside routine working hours.

One Burn's night, my wife and I were invited to supper at our church minister's home. He was proud of his Scottish ancestry and we had a memorable meal with scotch broth to start; haggis, tatties and neeps for the main course; then cheese and oatmeal biscuits to finish. Any whisky involved in the cooking was undetectable in this Presbyterian household, and no wee dram was on offer afterwards.

This turned out to be fortunate.

At about two o'clock in the morning, our phone rang and a doctor from the ward told me he was very worried about a child who had been admitted with severe diarrhoea, dehydration, and a temperature of 108 degrees Fahrenheit (42 Celsius). My immediate response was that this reading was mistaken. I had never encountered such a high temperature and was not even sure if the glass thermometer, then in use, read that high. He was agitated and insisted it was correct, making it clear the patient was very ill. I reassured him I would be there as soon as possible. I jumped out of bed and pulled on the clothes I had recently discarded. It was a bitterly cold January night but my elderly Ford, amazingly, started first time. As I accelerated away from home, I became aware of severe heartburn. My indigestion got worse throughout the 15-minute drive, not helped by the anxiety about what I might find when I arrived.

I cursed at every red traffic light, before screeching to a halt in front of the hospital. As I jogged up two flights of stairs to the isolation ward, acid regurgitated into my throat. I swore to myself never to eat haggis again. I continued at speed past the waiting junior doctor, and the nurses, into the ward kitchen. The night staff watched in disbelief as I downed a full pint carton of milk from the fridge. At last, relief! I would definitely avoid Burns suppers in future.

The poor child was very much worse than me, and indeed had an extremely high temperature. It was a little lower now as a result of a dose of aspirin and the application of cool cloths. She was a little delirious and therefore difficult to examine. Her tummy seemed tender when touched. There was the beginning of a rash on her skin. She was passing copious volumes of diarrhoea and her blood chemistry was consistent with considerable fluid loss. Correction would require careful fluid management, with close monitoring of her blood chemistry. This was the worst case of infective diarrhoea I had seen, and the little girl was ill out of proportion to the rotavirus gastroenteritis cases we commonly encountered. Her parents waited anxiously to hear my opinion. Worried myself, I phoned my consultant. I explained that something unusual was going on, and I would value the benefit of her expertise. I had learnt by now to know my limitations.

She came in straight away. I had the impression that she, too, had not seen this level of fever before. She calmly took charge and agreed we must take multiple cultures, not just of the diarrhoea fluid, but also of blood samples. We reviewed the abdominal X-ray, which was of little help. We explained to our staff that the little girl must be kept isolated and "barrier" nursed, i.e., attending staff should wear disposable gowns, masks and gloves, in order to prevent the infection spreading. We prescribed broad range antibiotics and appropriate intravenous fluids. We talked at length with the parents.

It was not yet dawn on the wintery morning as we left for home to shower and change our clothes before returning to work. My colleague's car sat next to mine in the almost empty staff car park. As she unlocked the door, she was greeted by a cacophony of barking.

"Well, doctor," she said, "at least I will have company on the way home."

She got in and started the engine. The rumour around the hospital that she kept five pet dogs was apparently true.

It was mid-morning when I had a call from our bacteriologist.

"These samples you sent in overnight, I am pretty sure they contain Salmonella typhimurium," he said.

"You mean the organism that causes typhoid fever?" I queried, almost disbelieving what he was telling me.

"Yes, your patient has typhoid, I'm afraid!"

I congratulated him on the speed of his diagnosis and, as I set off to find the boss, I was thankful I had spent some time washing before eating breakfast and had put my clothes into our antiquated washing machine before leaving home.

We adjusted the antibiotic treatment appropriately. Our girl, now better rehydrated, was much improved and more alert - although still extremely ill with a high swinging temperature. The parents were shocked by the news we delivered. We reassured them she was on the correct treatment and should be fine in a few days, as we set about questioning them about any unusual food or meals the family had recently eaten. They had never been abroad, they said - but unfortunately, they owned a greengrocer's shop.

The public health troops swung into action once we notified them. Over the next few days, unusually, there were several adults in the area also diagnosed with typhoid fever, but fortunately no more children. The family business was quarantined as a precaution. The source of the infection, however, was traced to a local Chinese takeaway, from which each victim had recently eaten food. I realised I too had eaten its food at least once, although without any ill effect. The problem apparently originated from a new cook recently arrived from abroad who was found to be an asymptomatic carrier of the typhoid bacterium. It closed down, never to reopen.

The child eventually made a full recovery - but later I learnt that, due to lack of customers, the family business had moved to another area of the city.

A worrying phone call

Another morning in the neonatal unit, as I checked a baby who was judged to be almost ready to go home, a nurse interrupted to deliver a message.

"I'm sorry, but there is a Sister Wallace on the phone. She is insisting you speak with her at once."

I was a little puzzled, as the only Sister Wallace I could think of was my old friend Wally from the adult medical ward, where I had worked a few years earlier. I wondered what she could want. I picked up the phone and said hello.

"Maurice, is that you?"

I recognised the voice at once. Somewhere in the back of my mind, it registered that she had not addressed me in her formal old school way as, doctor, but used my first name.

"Wally, it's a nice surprise to hear from you, how can I help you?"

There was a slight pause.

"Maurice, it's your father. He has just been admitted here, I'm afraid."

As I tried to take this information in, she spoke again.

"He's in no immediate danger, but he has had a stroke. The Professor has been with him and says everything is quite stable for now. His blood pressure is fine, and his heart is strong. There is some weakness down his right side and his speech is affected. Your mother is with him and is understandably quite upset."

Shaken, I stumbled out a reply.

"But, my dad is usually so fit. He rides a bike everywhere. He has never drunk alcohol or smoked. He has only just turned sixty."

I realised I was rambling and stopped. Sister Wallace spoke again.

"I know this is a terrible shock, but if you can get away, you should come over here as quickly as you can."

I was soon on my way, driving through the city traffic, wondering if things were more serious than Sister wanted to say on the phone. When I entered my father's side ward, directly opposite her office, dad smiled weakly and tried to speak but he couldn't find the words. He ended up shaking his head to tell me not to worry and gave me the thumbs up sign to say he was okay. His old skill with sign language, learnt long ago because both his parents had hearing difficulties, came in useful in this situation. He was pale and, despite all that had happened to him, tried to put on a brave face for us. I hugged this man I loved and turned to hug my mother as the tears welled in her eyes.

I sat talking and tried to reassure everyone by saying his speech and strength would probably recover in a few days. After a while, dad closed his eyes and drifted off to sleep. My mother said, "We will just have to trust in the Lord to bring him through."

I went to thank Wally and speak to a doctor.

Suddenly, my so-far relatively successful career as the first doctor in my family took on a new perspective.

My father did indeed slowly recover but it was a year before he was able to return to work. It was to be the first of several strokes which ultimately led to his early death at the age of 64 years. My mother outlived him by over twenty years. I cannot remember her complaining much about her own loss, which she felt keenly. It was years before she talked freely to me about her sorrow in those days. By then I knew she felt it was her husband, more than herself, who had been cheated.

A career determining encounter

In late summer, I was contacted by a local family doctor who had seen an eight-year-old girl with what appeared to be a peculiar allergy. Rachel had been brought to his surgery some weeks earlier with swollen eyes. He examined the child but found no rash or itch. Her mother was sure Rachel had not eaten anything different from usual. The family had a well-cultivated garden, where her father took pride in the display of flowers and shrubbery. In the warm August weather, the child had been playing outside with her friends for most of the day. The GP concluded she had hay fever with allergic conjunctivitis and prescribed antihistamines.

These proved ineffective and, on the third occasion that he saw Rachel, who continued to be otherwise well and energetic, her mother pointed out that now her ankles also seemed a little swollen. Since this was not a symptom he associated with simple hay fever, he requested a hospital opinion.

At the clinic visit, I heard that the swelling around her eyes was most obvious in the morning and almost disappeared by evening time. When examined, she had quite a big tummy - swollen, I suspected, with retained fluid. She did not actually appear unwell.

Every child who attended that clinic was routinely asked to pass a urine sample, irrespective of their symptoms. I had previously asked the nurses the reason for this unusual practice and been told, "It's because the boss says so."

On this occasion, the ritual provided me with another clue to the diagnosis. The urine analysis showed a large amount of protein present, when normally none should be detectable. I concluded that Rachel had a kidney disease called nephrotic syndrome - a condition in which plasma protein leaks through the kidney's blood filter, the glomerulus, which usually only allows water and waste products to pass out as urine. Low plasma protein levels result in fluid accumulating in subcutaneous tissue and eventually in the abdominal cavity, in advanced cases. The tissue swelling is generally in dependent areas of the body such as the legs, and is known as oedema.

When the kidney function tests came through, the results showed a low level of the protein Albumin in her blood, and confirmed the diagnosis. The girl was commenced on a course of steroid tablets, the first line of treatment for this condition. I reassured the family that, in most instances, this induced a remission and kidney function would return to normal. This treatment, which suppresses the immune system's attack on the kidney tissue, is not without side effects, however, and was discontinued two months later, when Rachel failed to respond. Diuretic medication, to make her pass more urine, reduced the fluid retention and the puffiness was controlled, but I knew we were, at best, only able to control the symptoms of the underlying condition.

As the months passed by, I saw that there was a slow deterioration in Rachel's kidney blood tests. My concern was that, if this continued over years, the kidneys might eventually fail. We introduced a more aggressive chemotherapeutic regimen. Cyclophosphamide was a more powerful drug in counteracting the underlying glomerulonephritis, but required weekly blood tests to monitor white blood cell levels and avoid a potentially dangerous side-effect of bone marrow suppression. Again, there was little response.

I knew that kidney dialysis treatment and kidney transplantation was now being performed in the nearby adult renal unit. Although our patient was nowhere close to needing such treatment, I inquired about the criteria for access to the programme. I learned that it was restricted to those between the ages of fifteen and 55, who had no history of heart disease, diabetes, tuberculosis or psychiatric illness.

I searched the medical literature in the hope of finding some alternative treatment which might arrest Rachel's condition. By chance, I came across information in *The Lancet* journal about a short course in London on renal disease in children. I mentioned it to my consultant, who shared my concern about our little girl. A short time later, she called me into her office to tell me that she had identified a hospital educational bursary which might pay for me to attend that nephrology course, if I was interested. She smiled, almost as pleased as me. We hoped I might learn of some innovative treatment to help Rachel.

Some months later, I sat in the lecture theatre at the Institute for Child Health, adjacent to the children's hospital at Great Ormond Street, for several days. I listened to talks on the most recent advances in the field. Lecturers from Europe and America shared their research and experience. I heard about recent advances in diagnosis and treatment and realised I had a lot yet to learn. However, there was nothing new which might arrest Rachel's condition. I was, however, alerted, to another condition called haemolytic uraemic syndrome, caused by a toxin produced by certain coliform bacteria. I realised I had seen a child with this condition without anyone then being able to put a specific name to the diagnosis. With empirical and supportive treatment that patient had recovered.

I discovered that, even at Great Ormond Street, the top paediatric centre in the country, there was no renal transplant programme. However, staff there were working closely with Guy's Hospital across London, where such a service had commenced with considerable early success.

The seeds had been sown for the future growth of my career.

A fright in our family

Treating seriously ill children on a daily basis makes one a more tolerant parent, grateful that your own are healthy. Even when my children were unwell, it was generally reassuring to be able to compare the difference between their condition and that of my hospital patients. My wife has been known to ask, "What do our children have to do to get an antibiotic?"

In the early summer of the year I travelled to London, shortly before we were due to set off on our first seaside holiday together, our one-year-old son seemed rather hot and out of sorts on awakening. We gave him a spoonful of paracetamol syrup but, a short time later, as he sat on the floor, suddenly he began to shiver and shake. Shocked and terrified that he would come to harm, we tried to act sensibly, despite our racing hearts. Anne's nurse training kicked in as she laid him on his side and held him gently in a safe position in case he vomited. His skin had become pale and his lips slightly blue. The duration of the shaking was short lived. To us, though, it seemed like an eternity before it subsided and I was able to examine him. I could see no obvious reason for his high temperature. We removed his clothes and sponged him with tepid water in an effort to cool him a little. He was sleepy now but managed a smile as if he was trying to help us keep calm. Shaken and worried, I phoned my consultant who lived nearby to ask if she would come to see him.

"Bring him straight to the hospital and I'll meet you in the infant ward," was her immediate reply.

We drove there, possibly ignoring the speed limit. My mind was racing over the various possibilities, although rationally I knew this was most likely just a rigor or simple febrile convulsion. These are not uncommon in older infants and toddlers who develop a high temperature with a viral infection. As we tore along the dual carriageway to the hospital, I told this to Anne. Perhaps I was also trying to convince myself and push the thought of meningitis from my mind.

We abandoned the car in the carpark and, carrying him, ran up the two flights of stairs to the ward. The doctor I had called was waiting and took over at once. In the clinical room, she examined him meticulously, as always. Still hot and miserable, he was taking an anxious interest in his surroundings. Wary of the strangers around him, he became very upset when a blood sample was taken. I tried to step back into the role of dad, rather than doctor. His crying reduced his mum to tears, but my senior colleague was reassuring.

"There are no signs of meningitis or of anything more serious," she said quite firmly.

"A lumbar puncture is not necessary but I want him to stay in hospital. I'm sending off blood and urine cultures and some other tests - and I expect they'll be normal. He's definitely got a nasty infection, probably viral, but I'm starting him on a course of intramuscular antibiotics as a precaution."

As she talked with us, the nurses were wrapping him in iced sheets on her instruction, which produced further upsetting howls of protest. It seemed like a form of torture. Despite my trust in the consultant's judgement, part of me wished she had performed the lumbar puncture, while another part did not want it to be done unnecessarily. I accepted that her antibiotic regimen would cover any serious bacterial infection, as proved to be the case. Mark hated the injections, of course. I never used ice to cool a conscious child again. Indeed, it is possible cooling the skin during a fever may actually cause the body's core temperature to rise. Regular administration of paracetamol suspension is much more effective, and this was proven when a missed dose allowed a spike in temperature and another brief episode of shaking. Thankfully, no bacteria were isolated from the blood and urine cultures. These negative results and the white cell analysis suggested there was most likely an underlying viral infection.

Although Mark was miserable with the infection and extremely upset each time he had an injection, his mum and one favourite nurse, Jan, could coach a smile from him as he gradually improved over the following week.

So it was that we spent our holiday in a children's ward, rather than by the seaside. We did not care about this when we took Mark home well and fully recovered. It took us a while longer to recover and catch up on lost sleep.

Forever after, I had a deeper understanding of the emotional roller coaster suffered by the parents of sick young patients. It also confirmed my view that parents are an essential presence in any treatment. Hugs and cuddles have considerable therapeutic power.

9. Extra responsibilities

"There are only two paediatricians and a couple of SHOs on the medical team in our hospital,'' the senior consultant explained on my arrival at my next posting on the registrar training rotation. He greeted me warmly and offered me tea, or coffee, with him and his colleague. As we sipped from our mugs, he continued briefing me. I was informed that there was a paediatric surgical Senior House Officer (SHO) who worked on an out-of-hours rota on site, with the two from the medical side. The two consultants worked alternate nights and weekends, covering the hospital from home.

There was a pause and the other consultant spoke up.

"We have been wondering how you would feel about working a one in three rota with the two of us, rather than with the junior staff?"

He paused, noting my body language.

"I realise this would be a bit of a jump in responsibility, but you have all the tickets for a consultant job and quite a bit of experience now. We would make sure one of us was around to back you up if you had any difficulties while you settle in. Would you at least think about it?"

I swallowed, flattered but apprehensive. The proposal seemed somewhat irregular, but I felt compelled to agree to a trial period of a few weeks. The challenge was daunting but ultimately irresistible to an ambitious registrar. Later, when the arrangement inevitably became permanent, it occurred to me that there had been no suggestion that I would be offered any remuneration at all for the extra night commitment and responsibility incurred.

After a couple of months, I found myself taking a particular interest in the Special Care Baby Unit referred to locally as the Sciboo. It was an enthusiasm I shared with one of my mentors. The day-to-day treatment of the preterm infants tested my practical skills, and presented me with new clinical problems to overcome. With time, I felt I was getting to a point where I could cope with most of their problems. Even these tiny infants, however, made sure I did not become over confident.

Not quite ready for the road

"I think it's maybe time we moved little Nicole into a cot for a few days and started to think about when you might be able to take her home. Do you agree?"

I stood, leaning back against the neonatal incubator, as I broke the good news to Frances and Glen. They made no effort to hide their delight. I was feeling rather pleased with their baby's progress myself.

"She's been a real little fighter and has come along so well. She hasn't had an apnoea attack for almost a week. Her breathing is easy and regular now. So we are almost there."

I had come to know this little family very well since their daughter arrived in the world, about six weeks ahead of schedule. Her initial trouble breathing had been overcome by delivering extra humidified oxygen into a clear plastic box placed over her head. This enriched atmosphere maximised her immature lungs' ability to absorb adequate amounts of oxygen. With less work required from her chest muscles, her breathing had become less laboured, preventing her from becoming exhausted. Gradually, we had been able to reduce the amount of supplemental oxygen she received, guided by monitoring its concentration in her blood until the readings remained normal when in ordinary room air. In those days, measuring her oxygen saturation required a blood test. Today, skin oximeters are clipped to a tiny toe, and calculate oxygen saturation by shining a beam of light through the blood. The amount of light absorbed varies directly in relation to the amount of oxygen carried in the blood haemoglobin. However, despite stable blood oxygen readings, Nicole decided to give us an extra scare.

Every so often, the immature respiratory control centre in her brain would forget to send the signals to her chest and lungs to breathe and the resulting pause, or apnoea, would trigger the respiratory monitor alarm. The experienced midwives had coped with this sort of problem before in many premature babies, and knew that a little external stimulus, usually a gentle finger flick to a tiny foot, was enough to cause an intake of breath. Nicole's breathing would then settle back into a regular rhythm. Her mum, who rarely left her side, also became quite proficient at this technique, impressively overcoming her initial fear and panic when Nicole held her breath. The episodes gradually became infrequent and stopped. By the time we spoke, the respiratory monitor had not been triggered for a couple of days. It was discovered years later that small amounts of caffeine could prevent these attacks, an effect similar to that of strong coffee stopping some adults from falling asleep. The proposed plan was that, once we were happy she was safe and content, nursed in a cot in the unit, we would suggest that her mum came back into hospital and looked after her on her own, in a side ward off the nursery, for a few days and nights. This was to build up the parents' confidence, so they would feel comfortable looking after her at home.

As I was talking to Frances, her happy smile suddenly vanished. "Doctor," she cried, "is she not having a little turn right now?"

I spun around. Nicole was indeed not breathing and her lips were a little dusky. I opened the incubator door and gave her a gentle shake and all was well again. I thanked the nurse who had rapidly appeared at my side with a resuscitation bag and mask.

"It's okay. Thankfully, we won't be needing that. I think she just wanted to tell us she needs to stay in her incubator a little longer," I said apologetically.

I checked the baby over carefully to be sure there was no sign of chest infection, or any other reason for this late episode.

Although this was a Sunday morning, instead of heading home as usual after my round, I stayed nearby catching up on paperwork for a while before checking on the baby again. I had learned to err on the side of caution with the tiny ones in my care.

Just over a week later, Nicole safely made the trip home, at last.

Chocolate cake for breakfast

Understaffing in the NHS is a not a new phenomenon and, in recent times, has generally been blamed on undoubted underfunding and the demands of an expanding elderly population, not to mention imposed government reorganisations, interference and incompetence. In the mid-1970s, when I was posted to a district general hospital serving 10 or more country towns and the surrounding rural farming community, with a population of around 300,000, the establishment of a paediatric hospital facility and the appointment of local paediatricians were major innovations. There was a

134

single combined medical and surgical paediatric ward, alongside the neonatal special care baby unit, where Nicole had been cared for. There was also a busy outpatient service, delivered in the base hospital and at two smaller outlying units. The development of a comprehensive province-wide paediatric service was in its infancy and possibly not considered a political priority. Most paediatricians were optimistic, overworked generalists, committed to a calling which they, like myself, considered to be a privilege. Only in the central university hospital were there individuals who had sub-specialty expertise in a few areas.

The consultants I worked with there became friends and, when one of us was on holiday, the other two absorbed their work -which, in my case, included being seconded to look after some peripheral clinics.

On the first occasion I arrived to undertake such a clinic at the small hospital some 20 miles away from base, I belatedly discovered on arrival that patients were booked to be seen for both a morning and an afternoon session. I soon realised that my speed at history-taking and diagnosis was not quite fast enough to permit a break for lunch. Instead, I was lucky to grab a cup of tea and a biscuit

My hunger was not improved by the first consultation of the afternoon.

I read the minimalist referral letter. "Obese child. Glandular basis?" was all it said.

"Your family doctor is concerned about your little girl's weight?" I ventured to her mother, who was rather rotund herself.

"Yes, but big bones run in our family and she is tall for her age," she countered.

The little girl's weight and height had been recorded by the clinic nurse.

"Let's just see where she is on this weight chart," I said, plotting her weight on the graph against her age. I slid the chart over so that the mum could see the lines marked on it and the dot I had added representing the patient.

"This is called a percentile chart. Only three children in a hundred would be below the bottom line on the chart; and only three would be above the top line. The weights of the other 94 per cent lie between the upper and lower lines," I explained.

I indicated where I had plotted her daughter's weight, well above the ninety-seventh percentile line for her age, suggesting Shirley was one of the top three by weight, out of one hundred children of the same age. As her mother studied the record, I chatted to the little girl, admiring the pretty dress she was wearing, her socks with frilly tops and her patent shoes. She smiled coyly. She was clearly a cherished child. We talked for a while about how she managed during school physical activities. Shirley volunteered that she very easily got short of breath and sometimes had to sit out. I nodded sympathetically. Apparently the family had wondered if perhaps she could have asthma. I readily agreed to have a listen to her chest but asked if it was possible that her limited exercise tolerance might be just because she was a little heavy. The mother looked sceptical.

"Just before I examine Shirley, can you tell me about her appetite? What would she eat for breakfast, for instance?"

"Well, she doesn't like cereal and I cannot let her go to school on an empty stomach."

" Mmm," I nodded noncommittally. "So what does she have instead?"

"Well doctor, the only thing she will eat in the morning is chocolate swiss roll."

I hid my surprise.

"She has a slice of a chocolate Swiss roll for breakfast?"

"No, not a slice."

"Ah - you mean those little individual Swiss Rolls? I understand they're very popular as treats."

Her mother began to look a little flustered.

"No doctor, a whole Swiss roll or I wouldn't be able to get her to go to school."

"So, she eats a complete chocolate cake for breakfast?!"

I was unable to hide my amazement now. The rest of her diet was equally bizarre. I did my best to treat both mother and daughter sympathetically. I arranged some thyroid and metabolic blood tests and a check of the child's blood sugar, which proved to be normal.

The mother probably knew what the problem really was, and without hesitation agreed to an appointment with a dietician. We did not have a psychologist available so I might have had to take on that role.

I was already behind, but the time spent taking a thorough history and winning the mother's cooperation was hopefully well spent. Childhood obesity is not new, just much more common in the twenty-first century.

The six o'clock call

Thankfully, neither patients nor staff complained as appointments ran late, perhaps tolerant of my youth. It was almost 6 p.m. by the time I saw the last child, put my feet on the desk and phoned Anne at home. Before I could explain she said, "You don't need to tell me. You are going to be late for dinner again". She referred to this as "the usual six o'clock phone call". I packed my bag, thanked the nurse who had volunteered to work late with me and headed for the car park. She called after me.

"Doctor, you do know they are expecting you up in the ward?"

"The ward?" I replied, astonished. "I only came to do the outpatient clinic."

"But the consultant always looks in on the patients the family doctors have admitted during the week," she explained.

Fortunately, there were only five or six children to be seen and none with any serious complaint. Indeed one was a nine year old boy whose only problem was persistent bed wetting at night. I doubted the training regimen he was prescribed for his hospital stay had any scientific basis. Some of the local general practitioners had admitting rights on the basis of some paediatric training and perhaps the possession of a diploma in child health. My input seemed to be more of a courtesy than a consultation, and I soon escaped.

I arrived home late in the evening, giving thanks that we did not have a dog who might have been given my dinner.

Reheated food had never tasted so good.

The modern hospital in which I found myself based was built to cope with the demands of an expanding population as part of an innovative urban plan. I enjoyed the work there and learned quickly to make decisions safely, in an environment where discussion and sharing problems was normal practice. There was a real team spirit in the children's wards, with less of the hierarchies entrenched in old traditional hospitals. Local nurses and other staff took great pride in their new hospital and the service they provided.

Two adjacent county towns, and the countryside between, were being redeveloped as a new city. Initially this was hoped to be an answer to the overcrowding and industrial decline of Belfast. It welcomed new people and new industries which were facilitated by generous government grants. In the early days, it had proven difficult to persuade families to move from their traditional big city enclaves to the new town and to the countryside. Gradually, people were attracted by the modern homes, traffic-free housing estates, new industries and jobs. Unique among the newcomers were Vietnamese boat people, refugees who had fled from the war which had raged in their homeland, and from the new regime which took control after the Americans left. Gradually, some diversity was creeping into the Northern Irish population. Others still had moved to the new development hoping to find respite from the violence of the divided big city.

Broken bones

"There's something on this chest X-ray which I needed to show you immediately."

The radiologist was speaking in front of the light box, which illuminated a film clipped to the screen. I stood behind him in the gloom of his darkened office, examining the image revealed.

"There's little evidence of infection in the lungs, but careful examination of the ribs reveals why this little boy may be having difficulty breathing." I focused my gaze on the right side of his chest, where the radiologist was pointing out cracks in three of the child's bones with the tip of his pen.

"Equally important are these small areas of calcification in two ribs on the left side, indicative of previous healed or healing fractures."

138

My heart sank, for I knew rib fractures in an infant were unlikely to be accidental.

Later in the day, I sat down in the ward office with a senior nurse and the child's parents. First we confirmed that their son was fine for now. He was not ill, his breathing was improving, and they had done the right thing by bringing him to hospital. Then came the difficult moment. I explained I had needed to talk with them urgently because of the changes we found on his X-ray. I went on to say that we had identified several rib fractures, which I offered to show them.

I withdrew the films from a large brown envelope.

"What I need to ask you," I said, "is if you have any idea how they might have happened?"

I watched their reaction carefully. They did not appear shocked. They were clearly uncomfortable and at a loss for words. The mother became upset, wiping tears from her cheeks. As the nurse offered her a box of tissues, she looked at her partner.

"He must have fallen or something," he volunteered. "Are you sure you couldn't be mistaken?"

"Let me show you the pictures. You will see there are two sets of fractures, as we can tell they happened at two separate times."

He stared at the pictures as I identified the breaks.

"Well, I just can't explain it," he said gruffly.

The mother nodded in agreement, looking down at her tightly clasped hands, without speaking.

I endeavoured to avoid making the meeting confrontational, and so went on to mention that there were babies with a rare condition called brittle bone disease, who could suffer hidden fractures. I explained we could see no evidence of that in their little boy - because in affected children, the whites of the eyes are instead blue. We planned, of course, to carry out more detailed tests, I said, but until we got to the bottom of this, I asked if they would agree for their son to be kept in hospital. I explained that I had a professional duty to look after his welfare. Indeed, if they were not agreeable, we would seek a legally-binding "place of safety" order to detain him.

I paused as they absorbed this information.

"If you have no questions, my advice, in the meantime, is for you to think again carefully about how he may have been injured. This is a difficult situation, and I am not blaming anyone for anything. My concern for now is for your little boy, but I have to inform you that the hospital social worker, and possibly the police, will wish to meet with you. I will be here and you can also talk to me, or one of my colleagues, at any time. I will help in any way I can."

I waited for a response and, receiving none, rose and offered my hand to each, to conclude the painful interview.

I was aware that the only people who were likely to know what exactly happened were the immediate family members. Innocent individuals may or may not have witnessed the violence; they may be unwilling to accuse the aggressor out of a false sense of loyalty; perhaps they were also a victim, or were afraid of becoming one. While it would be possible to protect the child through the courts, with a care order removing them from a dangerous situation, gaining a criminal conviction against the perpetrator would require the police to prove their case beyond reasonable doubt. This could be more difficult.

Northern Ireland was then a violent place with some 300 deaths each year due to the troubles. Within hospitals, conversely, we were dedicated to preserving lives. My experiences with political and sectarian atrocities reinforced my belief in non-violence. Even against this background, it was especially shocking to encounter domestic violence directed at children. I shared a repugnance of this, in common with all those nurses, doctors and other professionals who care for children. The custom of using the term "non-accidental injury," minimised the stark reality of child abuse. The government-promoted "Stranger Danger" campaign implied that depraved strangers were the main risk to children. People found it difficult to believe or admit the level of abuse within families. Meanwhile, abuse within the church and its institutions was hidden or ignored by those in authority and sexual abuse of children considered almost inconceivable. Times have changed, but it remains difficult for victims to speak and be heard.

On another occasion, a child was brought to the A&E department of one of the hospitals in which I worked, having allegedly suddenly become extremely unwell. The baby was gasping for breath, his blood pressure low, his pulse weak. In short, he was critically ill. Initially, his condition was thought to be due to sepsis, or maybe an overwhelming pneumonia. Despite treatment with intravenous fluids, antibiotics and aggressive resuscitation, the child died shortly after arrival. The resuscitation team were unclear about why the baby had become desperately ill so quickly. Was there some underlying problem they had failed to recognise? Unhappy to provide a death certificate without a clear diagnosis, permission for a post mortem was sought. The parents refused to allow this to be performed. Such was the concern about the sudden death that the situation was discussed with the coroner. He used his legal powers to order the post mortem, which then did not require parental consent. Grandparents arriving at the hospital on learning of the tragedy and, significantly, although visibly distressed, supported his decision. They insisted that the family also needed to know why exactly their grandchild had died. This initially defused a difficult situation between staff and parents.

A pathologist carried out a detailed post mortem the following morning. His initial findings were shocking. He had identified hidden internal injuries, including a haemorrhage on the brain surface and an associated hairline skull fracture. With a senior paediatrician, he took control of pursuing the necessary legal procedures surrounding a suspicious death. The police were informed of the post mortem and began an investigation. Over the succeeding days, they and their forensic team established how and where the injuries had occurred. The suspected perpetrator was arrested, charged and, in due course, convicted.

Everyone involved in the case was enormously upset by the harrowing affair. There was sadness for a tiny life snuffed out, mingled with sympathy for the innocent and distressed extended family, and a barely suppressed disgust at the violence behind the crime. I spent some time pondering what state of mind or personality would lead someone to harm a baby. I wondered what stress, addiction, flawed upbringing, emotional or mental issues could interfere with an individuals ability to cope, to the extent that it resulted in violence.

Children are my Heroes …

In the midst of dealing with such an awful event, thankfully, there were always other patients demanding care and attention, generally with families who displayed the power of parental love, a reparative distraction from what seemed to be an unanswerable question.

10. Legends

Dr William at the Black Swan

I was surprised one evening to be contacted by a local family doctor who had a practice not far from our home. His name was unfamiliar to me. My caller, having explained who he was, suggested that I just called him "Dr William."

"Everyone calls me Dr William, and my wife, who shares the practice, is known by everyone locally as Dr Mary.

"We've been here a long time," he added. It was clear that he assumed I would know of him, but being new to the area, we had signed up with another general practice in the village, assuming it was the only one.

I was intrigued by his gentle, old-world manner. He went on to explain that he was looking for a reliable young person to look after his practice for a week, and that I had been recommended by a friend. I explained this would be almost impossible, since I had a full-time commitment at the hospital. He was not to be put off, however, and informed me that he'd obtained my phone number from the consultant physician for whom I was then working. This was another surprise, as I had assumed our bosses had no idea of - and indeed would have disapproved of - junior staff taking outside work. Perhaps my consultant had noticed my rather battered, second-hand Renault Four motor car, which even my wife unkindly referred to as "the trolley bus".

He insisted that he would really like to meet me, and suggested I might oblige him with a visit some evening, at least for a chat. Reluctantly, I agreed, feeling it would have been discourteous to refuse.

As I parked my old red car outside his house and made my way up the short drive to the beautiful detached Victorian property, I noted the polished brass plaque at the entrance, the immaculately kept gardens and the beautiful copper beech trees. I pressed the doorbell. Distantly, I could hear soft musical chimes. A trim white-haired gentleman in a three-piece suit opened the door and beamed at me, holding out his hand. "Dr William," he announced, stepping back to reveal Dr Mary, to whom I was introduced. Soon. I was sitting in the study, sipping tea with my hosts, who I reckoned were probably in their seventies. They made fascinating company. Rather than interview me, they reminisced about setting up the practice when they were my age, in the days before the NHS was introduced in 1948. Their warmth, enthusiasm and charm were already thwarting my plan to quickly and apologetically refuse the request, which I was sure would again be delivered.

I was intrigued by the history of their practice, learning they had originally chosen to settle in the village because it was then in the countryside outside, but close to, Belfast - although cut off from the city conurbation by fields and farms. With the passage of time, what was once a rural idyll had gradually been enveloped by urban sprawl.

Anne and I now lived in one of these newer developments. I learned the practice we'd signed up to had also been around for generations, passing down from father to son, creating a mini medical dynasty. Also, not fully aware of this history, Dr William and Dr Mary had bought the house in which we were now sitting and "put up their plate" on the wall beside the front door. As newcomers, however, they had faced great difficulty in attracting patients and almost lost hope of ever being accepted into the community. Then, one Saturday evening, their bell rang repeatedly, accompanied by a hammering at the door. They could hear raised voices. They rushed to answer and discovered two agitated men outside.

"Can you come quickly? Old Sam the butcher has been taken of a seizure and collapsed in the backyard of the Black Swan," they begged.

They didn't mention that they'd already discovered the other doctor was not at home.

Dr William grabbed his bag and ran 400 metres to the pub. A crowd had gathered, but parted as the young doctor pushed his way through to the yard, which housed the outside toilet. Sam, a well-known local character, was lying on the floor there, jerking, writhing and making incoherent noises. Dr Mary took up the tale.

"William knelt down beside him and quickly established he was still breathing. He could see that he was still a reasonable colour, somewhat the worse for drink, but actually in no immediate danger. He took out his stethoscope to check Sam's heart. Of course, to get at his chest meant unbuttoning his tight tweed waistcoat and shirt."

She paused.

"And then he was able immediately to identify the problem," she said, laughing at the memory,

"He knew exactly what he needed to do. He opened his medical bag wide, withdrew his case of instruments, opened it on the ground beside him, and selected a silver metal scalpel and forceps. At this, the crowd drew back, and so did not see William, dodging the flailing arms and legs, grasp a waistcoat button with the forceps and sliced the thread behind it with the scalpel. Sam had apparently fastened the button to his trouser flies, making him unable to straighten up. In his inebriated state, he had probably fallen over and was unable to rise, no matter how hard he struggled. Once released, he sprung up and, grasping his saviour by the arm, used his support to stagger to the bar and order them both a glass of Guinness Stout."

Dr William then added: "Many's a version of Sam's miraculous recovery circulated for months in the village and around about. Of course, neither Sam nor I revealed the true nature of the operation," he smiled, tapping his nose with a finger. "Professional confidentiality, you know?"

This event was a turning point for the couple, and the patients it attracted ensured their financial survival.

After an entertaining half-hour, I was unable to refuse being shown around the consulting room, waiting room and pharmacy, all of which were part of the family home. It was the typical old-style practice, familiar from my childhood, when the GP was a family friend as well as the family doctor. This ambience and the sense of professional tradition had strong appeal, but it was the story of old Sam and the button flies that made me have a change of heart and agree to use up a precious week of holiday and take up their offer.

One event during that week characterises for me the role of the family doctors of that generation. Each morning, before and during the hours when I would see patients, the housekeeper and receptionist, Miss Primrose, answered and recorded telephone calls from people wishing to have an appointment or a home visit. Such visits were relatively common and there were often five or six required each day. When there were fewer, Miss Primrose explained to me that there was a list of elderly patients who the doctors visited in rotation, when they had time. I was shown a book that indicated the next person who might benefit from such a visit. No request was necessary. Here was an example of preventative medicine in action. A service impossible today in an overstretched, underfunded NHS. Once again, I was impressed. But there was more to come. One morning she asked me, "Did you listen to the morning news on the local radio?"

The station had been on in our kitchen, but I had not given it much attention. She continued, "You may have heard the tragic story of the police constable who was chasing a burglar last night, when he collapsed with a heart attack and died?" I vaguely remembered the story, heard against the background of a noisy family breakfast.

She handed me the list of home visits for the day and a second sheet of folded notepaper.

"I have written down the policeman's name and home address for you."

I was a little confused.

"I know that if Dr William or Dr Mary were here, one of them would call with the family. They always call with the family of any our patients who pass away, no matter what the circumstances."

I was rather taken aback but took the note and, after completing the other visits, drove to the constable's house, uncertain as to what I would say or do. I rang the doorbell, and it was opened by a woman whose eyes were red from weeping.

"Hello, I'm filling in for Dr William and Dr Mary while they're on holiday." I explained. "I've just called to offer my sympathy and see if there's anything I can do to help."

The door opened wide.

"Come in doctor," said the woman, taking my hand.

"We have been waiting for Dr William. We knew he would call. Thank you for coming."

146

Soon, I was sitting with a cup of tea in the family circle, listening to stories of the policeman as a son, husband and father. Later, as I took my leave, I asked again if there was anything else I could do to help. They felt no need for sleeping tablets, so instead I wrote down my home phone number, and assured everyone they could contact me at any time.

Regretfully, by the time I recognised it fully, I was too late to tell my mentors how much, in absentia, their holistic approach influenced my subsequent career and practice.

A country legend and the gunman

My final venture into general practice was a few years later in a small market town. The central square was dominated by a magnificent church. Hidden behind it, in a terrace of once-gracious town houses, was the doctor's surgery. It mainly served the surrounding farming community and traditional townsfolk, rather than the nearby new housing developments. I had, by then, completed my basic paediatric training, and so I was happy to undertake a week's attachment there, relieving one of the older partners. I had met Dr Davey on the ward where I worked, in the course of his unique habit of visiting any of his patients who were admitted to the hospital. I was to discover he was regarded with respect by his colleagues - and with a degree of awe by his patients.

My first morning taking his surgery passed without incident, and I joined the other staff for coffee, or more likely tea, in a little kitchen at the rear of the old house. The clinical rooms inside the entrance had been modernised and a faint whiff of antiseptic hung in the air. The rear had changed little over many decades, and reminded me of my grandmother's home when I was a child. I was made welcome in the tearoom, and even allocated my own mug. The nurses and receptionist set about weighing up the young newcomer. Strangely, I cannot recall other doctors being present, although I'm sure this was not a single-handed practice.

Pleased to discover that I had acceptable family connections in the town, they were soon offering helpful advice and I felt safe enough to confess that I hoped I could live up to the senior partner's reputation.

"Well," one of the district nurses remarked, "sometimes he does things in his own unique way, so I wouldn't concern yourself too much. Just you do things the right way and you'll be fine." Wise counsel offered.

Later in the week, when Iwas feeling more at ease with the staff, I asked what exactly this comment had meant. Various examples were given, mainly along the lines that he didn't rush to refer people to the hospital or casualty, but preferred to rise to the clinical challenge and successfully treat patients himself, if at all possible. My impression was that this also meant he was prepared to perform minor surgery and treat the sort of trauma sustained by farm workers on the premises, without recourse to unnecessary investigations, relying rather on his own diagnostic skill, which seemed to be infallible. Eventually, I was asked if I had not heard about how he had once faced down a gunman and disarmed him.

"He did what?" I asked in disbelief.

"You've probably noticed the police station on the other side of the square?" came the answer. This would have been impossible to miss as, like most police buildings in Northern Ireland at that time, it was encased in a heavy wire mesh cage, rising higher than, and sloping over, its roof. The metal poles supporting this framework were embedded in enormous concrete blocks. This ugly facade was designed to stop car bombs and mortar or rocket attacks destroying the station and the officers inside.

It was at this police station where the dramatic story of the gunman unfolded. One day, an agitated woman came running through the front door of the surgery shouting, "Is Dr Davey here?"

The doctor stepped out of his room to find out what all the commotion was about. In a panic, the woman said a young man, armed with a gun, had managed to force his way into the station and was threatening to kill everyone inside. She had been at the counter in the entrance hall, talking to a constable who was (thankfully) behind a pane of bullet proof glass, trying to sort out a minor traffic offence, when the gunman arrived. He was not interested in her and so, terrified, she had fled past him and made her escape. The assailant was now in a stand-off with the police, who remained behind the armoured internal doors. She was convinced that, sooner or later,

148

someone would get shot or injured and ran to the surgery to pre-emptively find a doctor.

I heard how he instinctively grabbed his medical bag and, without further thought, rushed to the station, shouting out his name and profession as he entered (doctors, priests and clergy still had a strange immunity in those violent days).

He immediately identified the young man who, on recognising the face of his family doctor, was momentarily distracted. Dr Davey strode over to him, telling him that he had delivered him at birth, knew who he was, and knew his mother. He snatched the gun out of the young man's hands before he could recover from this unforeseen intervention, scolding him that his mother, a good woman, would be ashamed to know what he was up to. Another nurse intervened to claim that the doctor had told the agitated young man that he'd helped bring him into the world and had no desire to see him leave it again. The situation was defused, no-one was injured and the story, based on fact (although possibly embellished) , entered the mythology of those troubled times.

Fortunately, I did not have to deal with any such dangerous situations during my short period as his replacement - but can bear witness to the good doctor's occasionally unusual methods. He had left a request, for instance, for me to check on an elderly lady who, being of limited mobility, had fallen after becoming a little light-headed, sustaining a broken arm and some other, more minor, injuries. I parked my car on the roadside near a muddy lane leading to her whitewashed cottage. Tramping up to the door, my enjoyment of the countryside and birdsong was ruined as my best shoes sank into the mud and cow clap splattered the trousers of my only suit - compulsory dress locally for someone in my profession. I cleaned my feet as best as I could before entering a living room so spotless that I felt I should remove my filthy footwear, and maybe leaving it to dry in front of the roaring fire.

I was led upstairs by the lady's daughter to a bedroom where the white-haired matriarch sat queen-like, propped up on pillows, with a quilted bed jacket, rather than ermine, draped around her shoulders. Her view out the facing window was across green fields with Lough Neagh in the distance. Her right arm, encased in plaster of Paris, was resting on a pillow by her side.

Her daughter fussed about, straightening the patchwork quilt and tidying magazines away. I introduced myself and explained I had come to check on her arm and her injuries. Her main interest was in gaining my permission to be up and out of bed again. Her daughter raised her eyes heavenward. I asked what advice she had been given by the hospital about this.

"Hospital?" she said, bemused. "I have never been near a hospital in my life and don't intend to start at my age!"

Wondering which of us was more confused, I asked how, if this was the case, she had had the fracture set and the plaster applied.

"Old Davey could teach you young lads a thing or two," she said, nodding and smiling

"He summoned the midwife, along with her gas and air machine and she held the mask over my face. It made me feel right funny, and I must have fallen asleep for a minute, but when I started to come around, he was taking wet plaster of Paris bandages out of a basin, borrowed from our kitchen, and wrapping them around my arm. He held my hand in a vice-like grip and wouldn't let me move the arm for a good 15 minutes before putting it in a sling when the plaster had set. I hardly felt a thing."

On inspection, the plaster was perfect, the arm straight, and she demonstrated that she could wiggle her fingers. I measured her blood pressure in bed. Then we helped her up and into a chair, where I checked her blood pressure again. It was steady. Now reassured, she wanted to get downstairs. I suggested perhaps that should wait until the next day, providing she was able to walk to the tiny bathroom without becoming dizzy or falling again. She seemed satisfied - but I left feeling my advice did not carry the same weight as that of the man who could set broken bones anywhere.

Another visit was with a farmer. Again, he was of that generation who avoided doctors if possible. Although still active about the farm, the family business was now run by his son. His wife had called in on his behalf to request some liniment that would reduce the swelling which had developed in his ankles. He had been offered an appointment to see the doctor, who explained that rheumatic embrocation was unlikely to solve the problem, since both ankles had swollen, and neither had been hurt nor twisted. The farmer then took over the phone himself and suggested the provision of some strong crepe bandages to bind his ankles, suggesting this might work. Dr Davey repeated that he needed to come in to be examined, saying the patient's proposed approach would, at best, merely mask the problem. The farmer insisted that he was perfectly well. It was just that his large ankles meant he couldn't get his boots on and get about his work. This story had been relayed to me at a hand-over meeting. In exasperation, the patient was advised that he had two options, to come in and be seen, or to cut down and widen the sides of his work boots.

Of course, this latter advice had not been meant to be taken seriously. A week later, I was on my way to see him because he had become quite short of breath when he tried to do any work, and the swelling was worse. In fact, when I got there, he was actually in bed, because any exertion exhausted him.

I concluded he had a degree of heart failure and, after percussing his chest with my fingers and listening with my stethoscope, suggested there was fluid collecting at the base of his lungs. He denied ever having any pains in his chest and was unwilling to believe his symptoms were due to a problem with his heart. I was faced with a country man who refused to go to hospital, yet I couldn't leave him without treatment. I insisted on giving him an injection of diuretic to cause him to pass increased quantities of urine, and started him on low doses of a drug to increase the strength of his heart. He accepted these reluctantly.

I spent 30 minutes with his son and wife, trying to impress on them that a hospital referral was imperative, while awaiting the response to the intravenous shot. He was in the toilet twice before I left, and his breathing had possibly improved, so I provided extra doses of the same drug, to be taken by mouth each morning and early evening. I called back after evening surgery, and daily thereafter, until my tenure was up. By then, he had agreed to be seen by the local cardiologist and the family guaranteed he would not miss the urgent appointment I had arranged. On my final visit, he was up and about, no longer short of breath but banned from any strenuous exercise. As we shook hands, he said to me: "You can tell that old git Davey that he owes me a new pair of work boots."

11. A Christening

After several years of hospital experience, I decided it was time to apply for the final step on the training ladder. I felt uncertain, in the face of stiff competition, that I would be successful. My intuition proved to be unreliable and I gained the title of Senior Registrar, one step away from becoming a tenured consultant. Before I was long in the post, I realised that with it came new and unexpected demands and responsibilities.

Late one evening, I walked briskly through a light drizzle towards the maternity hospital building. I had been presented with an unusual request and, oblivious of the rain, was pondering how I would cope with it. I donned a clean white coat and entered the neonatal ICU. Sister came quickly to brief me as we walked past a row of incubators and introduced me to the parents of a frail, very premature infant who was not responding to intensive treatment for sepsis. After shaking their hands, I explained I was the senior paediatrician in the hospital that night and had come to help in any way I could.

"We're afraid our baby won't survive the night. We know everything possible has been done for her, but she's slipping away," the father told me, trying to keep his voice steady. His wife continued, "We're anxious to have her baptised while she's still with us, but the nursing staff haven't been able to contact the hospital chaplain. We phoned our own priest, but he's already out visiting an ill elderly parishioner and he is fifty miles away."

She looked at her husband, "We would be very grateful if you would Christen our baby girl."

Sister had already told me about this request. I had no experience of the Catholic sacrament of baptism but I knew it was extremely important to those of that faith.

A midwife appeared at the edge of my vision and shook her head discreetly. I understood this to confirm that, yet again, there was no response from a priest. I had been reassured by the Sister that doctors had stood in for the clergy before in this situation. I learned from her that anyone can baptise a baby in an emergency, even someone who is not baptised themselves.

I spoke with the parents for a few minutes about what they had been through and reassured them that, of course, I was more than willing to do what they asked. I explained gently that this was not something I had done before. I just needed a couple of minutes to prepare.

I was still trying to think of a suitable form of words. I rehearsed my suggestions with Sister and was reassured by her advice.

My throat constricted with the emotion of the moment. I sipped a glass of water to loosen it up. Then I returned to talk again with the mother and father about the battle their little girl had fought, attempting to understand how they felt, before I confirmed the name they had chosen.

Sister joined us, bringing a vial of sterile water previously blessed by the hospital's Catholic chaplain. She poured this Holy Water into a small plastic receptacle. In the background, the bright lights and the sound of the monitors seemed to fade.

Sister opened the side of the incubator and a port on the opposite end. The baby's mother held one of her daughter's tiny hands and her father the other. Most of the nurses gathered around. I could almost feel another presence around us.

I dipped my fingers in the water and closed my eyes briefly.

"Dear Lord, take this little one into your loving care," I prayed, dribbling a little water onto her head.

I made the sign of the cross with my wet fingers on her forehead.

"I baptise Mary in the name of The Father, The Son, and The Holy Spirit."

We stood in silence for a few moments. The parents sobbed as we closed the incubator doors, then tried to smile. Sister hugged them both. She offered them a cup of tea, but they shook their heads and sat down to continue their silent vigil.

As they sat there, I stood behind them for several minutes, a hand on each of their shoulders. Mary's father turned around.

"Thank you, doctor," he said, as his wife nodded and tried to smile.

"This has been a very special privilege for me. Thank you for allowing me to do this for you and for Mary. It's something I will never forget."

Keeping focus

The promotion had brought me back to work in the academic unit of the major regional hospital. Inevitably, my thoughts returned again to the girl with failing kidneys, who I had encountered several years before in another hospital. I had tried to keep in touch and follow her progress over the years and concluded that her outlook had not improved. Now, as a senior registrar, I wanted to find a way to specialise in nephrology. My ultimate aim was to develop a dialysis and kidney transplant service for children, similar to the provision already in place for adults.

On Wednesday mornings, I shared an outpatient clinic with the Professor and sometimes joined him for coffee or lunch in the canteen. On one of these occasions, he informed me that the neurologist from the adult side of the hospital, who consulted on difficult or unusual cases in his area, was planning to retire in two or three years.

"We will need to prioritise training someone to replace him," he added meaningfully.

He elaborated at length, before we discussed some of the children we had seen that morning - as well as more mundane matters like the recent international rugby and football games. I realised he had raised the neurology topic to pique my interest. I had a dilemma, as I needed his support to further my future plans, which lay in a different direction altogether. I agreed with his thinking regarding the need for paediatric sub-specialists but avoided mentioning my personal interest at that point. When talking to other younger consultants about my ambitions, I inevitably found myself recounting the story of Rachel's plight and advocating the need for a renal replacement service for children. My aspiration gradually became general knowledge - although not, as yet, supported as a local priority.

A few months later, at coffee again, but now feeling more confident, I broached the subject of sub specialising in kidney disease with the Professor. By then, he was aware that I was not interested in a post in neurology and had identified another candidate. We discussed how difficult it might be to gain the necessary expertise in my proposed field. I explained my motivation to him and received a sympathetic hearing. He pointed out it would be necessary to persuade the local Department of Health and the

Postgraduate Medical Training Council of the need for a paediatric nephrologist. They held the budget for service development and for specialist training, respectively.

Having been challenged to think about how I might do this, I set about developing a strategy and a sound argument, based on reliable evidence, to underpin my proposition. It would take more than the story of one unfortunate child.

I explored the hospital database for information. It was held on card index files that recorded each admission by diagnosis. Computerised digital systems were far in the future. It took months of laborious work in the dusty records offices, where the clerical staff were pleased to welcome the rare appearance of a doctor. They were interested in my research and keen to hear about some of the patient's stories that were spurring me on. With their help, I was able to identify more than 500 patients admitted with kidney conditions over the previous five years. These accounted for four per cent of all admissions. This number did not include those who only attended as outpatients, as there was no diagnostic record available for them. There were also patients with renal complaints seen at nearby children's units, who were not included in the figures.

I obtained permission to invite a sample of patients from the five-year period to return for a follow-up assessment as part of a research project.

No child with advanced renal failure was listed - possibly because they were not referred, in the knowledge that no further treatment was available. I identified a small number who had conditions which were likely to deteriorate to the end stage of renal failure, when dialysis and transplantation would become the only hope for long term survival. A significant group had inherited conditions, and of these some undoubtedly had adult family members who were already in advanced renal failure, or who had died as a result of the condition. There were children born with spina bifida who had associated poor bladder function due to damaged nerve supply. Inadequate bladder emptying predisposes these patients to frequent urine infections and possible kidney damage.

I discovered that fewer than 10 percent of the hundreds identified had ever had their blood pressure recorded, despite renal conditions being the most common cause of high blood pressure in children. Controlling hypertension is a key factor in delaying deterioration in damaged kidneys.

I proceeded to present my findings at clinical research and education meetings, and to publish my findings in the local medical journal.

Permission to proceed

One afternoon, the professor called me into his office, where he sat comfortably behind a large mahogany desk. He smiled and asked me to pull up a seat. When I had settled, he went on to say that, at a dinner a few evenings earlier, he happened to be seated next to Dr McGeown, the head of the adult renal unit. He mentioned my ambitions and arguments for developing a renal service for children to her. Apparently, she had given my view her support and suggested I might like to join the large ward round she held each week. He had accepted on my behalf.

I was, of course, delighted and now knew I had won his support. Over succeeding months, I learnt a lot of practical nephrology from this national, indeed international, expert in the field. Many years later, she confided in me that, at my age, her ambition was to become a paediatrician - but that she had been informed by the then Professor that there was no position for a married woman in the Children's Hospital. As a result, she followed a different (and outstanding) career, her abilities having been recognised by other, more enlightened, physicians.

I was determined to build on the experience gained from adult nephrology and looked back at the details of the course I had attended in the Institute of Child Health and The Hospital for Sick Children in London. I wrote to the current course organiser, outlining the position in Belfast and seeking advice on how best I might train to fill the service deficiency. I received a brief reply from Professor Barrett suggesting that the next time I was in the capital, I should meet with him to discuss possible options. Of course, I was rarely in London but I immediately contacted his office and identified a mutually suitable date to visit some weeks later.

In the meantime, I continued my general paediatric work, gaining wider experience, facing new challenges, and learning my craft.

The baby at the gate

There are, of course, lighter moments working in paediatrics. The Royal Belfast Hospital for Sick Children, part of the Royal Victoria Hospital complex, faced onto the Falls Road, which is the main thoroughfare running several miles from the centre of the city to the housing estates on the outskirts of West Belfast. The nearby junction with the Grosvenor Road was known as "hijack corner" during the years of civil unrest, because of the number of cars which on stopping at the traffic lights were commandeered by gunmen or by scarey gangs of joy riders. A three-metre-high brick wall separated the hospital buildings from the busy road for many years. Throughout my time as a junior doctor, there was an open gate in the wall, immediately opposite the old hospital entrance. This gave easy and rapid access to the accident and emergency and outpatient departments, just inside. The locals also used this opening to walk to other parts of the complex, such as the adjacent Royal Maternity building, or as a short-cut to the lower Grosvenor Road, leading to the city centre.

At some point in the mid 1970s, an unidentified member of the site management decided this gate should be locked. Initially, this only happened when dusk fell. Admittedly the road was not always a safe place after dark, and joyriders were known to steal cars from the hospital car parks and race them up and down the Falls Road, challenging the police to intervene in what was, for them, a relatively no-go area.

Nevertheless, people from miles around continued to arrive at the gate with sick or injured children, as they and their parents had done for more than 40 years since the hospital opened. As I have mentioned, I myself had even been carried through it to the Emergency Department opposite, after a bicycle accident.

But now, families were being directed to proceed along the road, take a left turn at the traffic lights, follow another road to the hospital's rear entrance, before coming back up along the internal hospital road to arrive where they had started, but on the opposite side of the wall. When they at last entered the building, they passed the unfortunate security guard who had sent them off on this mile-long diversion. The edict was not universally popular with the local members of the public, nor with many staff. It was greeted with even less enthusiasm by the security staff, who had a small wooden hut near the gate, and were faced with distressed and angry parents pleading to be admitted. Some were sympathetic and may have even disobeyed instructions not to unlock the gate, but this risked putting their jobs on the line

One member of the hospital staff, also a local resident, observing the grief caused to families and the security staff, instigated a devious plan to draw attention to this inequitable situation.

Dressing up as a young woman, her face hidden in a headscarf, she approached the gate carrying a baby wrapped in a blanket in an apparent state of panic. She called out in a falsetto Belfast accent, frantically demanding to be let through. On being given the usual advice she became more upset and distressed, but the gate remained closed. The security guard tried to explain again as the shouting became almost hysterical, until she screamed, "Okay, here then, you take the baby into casualty and I'll run around the block."

She threw the baby still wrapped in a blanket over the gate. Miraculously, the guard caught the bundle - which in fact contained a small toy doll. By the time he recovered from the shock and realised he had been duped, the mother had vanished.

The story spread throughout the complex and, in the retelling, the doll often became an actual baby.

The prank was as unnerving for the security man as it was amusing for his colleagues, but sadly it had no impact on the administration. The gate remained closed until the wall was demolished, many years later, and replaced by a more pleasing metal railing, artistically constructed to represent the DNA double helix. A pedestrian opening was included but, by then, a new Accident and Emergency department had opened as part of a redevelopment of the hospital, and it was no longer near the main road.

12. Meeting the motorbike man

On the day I travelled to London, I stepped off the Piccadilly Line train at Russell Square station, and squeezed into one of the lifts, crushed against 20 or 30 other people. The metal doors slammed shut and we ascended to street level, where I was carried to the ticket barrier by the throng and expelled onto the street. I orientated myself and tried to avoid looking like a lost tourist. I turned right, then right again and was relieved to recognise the Institute of Child Health, with the famous Great Ormond Street Hospital for Sick Children behind. I had left Belfast on the morning London flight. Dressed in my only suit, and carrying a slim briefcase, I probably looked like one of the many business commuters.

I concentrated on walking confidently as I approached the entrance to the university. I was early for my mid-day appointment but remembered from my previous visit that there was a restaurant on the basement level of the building.

Entering, I was greeted from behind the reception desk by a rotund, uniformed man. I returned his "good morning," with a smiling "hello," and tried to continue on past, but he asked in a central European accent, who I was there to see. I later learned that he prided himself on knowing every doctor and scientist in the institute and, where possible, the ins and outs of their business.

"I have an appointment with Professor Barratt," I explained

"Nephrology and immunology," he acknowledged.

As he walked out from his office to meet me in the foyer, I noticed his pronounced limp. My glance turned out to have been rather obvious, and he immediately explained that his faltering steps were the result of a World War II wound, sustained when he was fighting with the Free Polish Forces. He offered me his hand, which I shook.

"You'll be coming to join us then?" he nodded knowingly. He was an expert at extracting information. He quickly learned that I was a doctor from Ireland and had almost an hour to kill. He confirmed that the coffee downstairs was good and told me the location of the Professor's laboratories.

We were now friends and confidantes.

I passed the time trying to read a newspaper. Eventually, I took the lift to the first floor, avoiding further inquisition. I knocked on the departmental office door. A distracted secretary answered and suggested I took a seat in the corridor, as the Professor had not yet arrived. Some time later, as I was debating whether I should knock again, she appeared wearing an outdoor coat. She informed me her boss should not be long and disappeared down the stairs.

I felt rather conspicuous as busy people constantly passed by, many in white lab coats. Several times, I felt them glance at me discreetly. It reminded me of sitting outside the Headmaster's study, after some misdemeanour.

Shortly after one o'clock, a youngish man approached with dishevelled long hair, dressed in full denim, and carrying a motorbike helmet.

"Are you waiting for someone?" he asked, with a peculiar twitch of his lips before he spoke. I explained again that I had an appointment with the Professor.

"Why don't you come in and have a coffee with me?" he suggested, as he pushed a door open. I followed and watched as he boiled a kettle and asked me about my journey, why I had come, and what my future plans were. Soon, I was talking about the child with kidney failure, whose future was bleak due to the lack of a paediatric renal service in Northern Ireland. I found myself telling someone other than my wife that I was determined to do something to correct this deficiency. I was encouraged by his lack of surprise at this aspiration and expanded. I explained that I needed to gain expertise in dialysis for children and, having attended a nephrology conference organised by Professor Barratt, I had arranged to meet him and seek his advice.

He must have noticed that I kept looking at the door, and said casually with a slight smile, "By the way, I should have introduced myself. I am Martin Barratt."

He waved away my apology and continued our talk. This gentle, astute man absorbed everything I said and responded as if we were equals. He was not how I had imagined the pre-eminent authority on Paediatric Nephrology in the country might be. My early experience of most consultants had generally been of rather distant, authoritarian figures, who dressed in three-piece suits with club or college ties tightly knotted in their shirt collars.

Paediatricians here were a different breed, it seemed.

After 40 minutes had flown by, he asked, "Would you like to come and meet some of my friends?"

Among those I met were Vanita Shah, his research scientist, and Dr Michael Dillon, another senior renal specialist. He and Professor Barratt discussed how they might help me pursue my dreams and ambitions, this time over a cup of tea. They came up with a proposal.

"We think your best option is to apply for a Medical Research Council training fellowship. If you're successful you could come and join the research team here and, at the same time, gain clinical experience in the hospital as an honorary registrar in the renal unit."

I was stunned and delighted. Had I somehow passed the initial interview?

Next, we discussed research areas I might explore. I explained that I had recently established the range of kidney diseases that affected children in Belfast and mentioned some ideas I'd formed. Mike Dillon seized on one suggestion. This was a tentative theory relating to kidney damage following urine infection in small children, which was the commonest problem identified by my research in Belfast. It was in keeping with some ideas which he was already exploring. He proposed that I flesh out my thoughts and put them in writing for them to review. He assured me they had considerable potential and he would be happy to advise me on how best to include them with the application. They were convinced that the case for training in dialysis and transplantation was self-evident. Should I be fortunate enough to be shortlisted, they would arrange for me to return and spend a day brainstorming with their team in preparation for the interview, which was the final stage of the application process.

I left an hour or two later, drained, inspired and exhilarated.

I called Anne from a phone box to report on my experience. She shared my excitement. I then had a chat with our two-year-old about his day. It seems his had been almost as exciting as mine - and much less stress free. He had been to a favourite park after seeing all his friends at nursery. On the journey back to Heathrow, I pondered on this new term I'd learnt - brainstorming.

Over the next few months, Dr Dillon and I developed a research plan exploring the mechanism which causes some children whose kidneys are scarred due to urinary infection to develop premature hypertension. Then, to my delight, a letter arrived inviting me to attend for a competitive interview at the Medical Research Council. The day before this, at The Institute for Child Health, I faced a group of scientists, researchers and doctors including Dr Dillon and Professor Barratt. I made a presentation, giving my reasons for applying for the fellowship and outlining my research proposal. I was hammered with probing questions, some supportive, some aggressive. There was a pause after any answer on which I stumbled, in which the interrogators were invited to offer advice and suggestions as to how I might make a more erudite response. On the morning of the interview, I spent an hour with a medical statistician, discussing how best the results of my study should be analysed.

When the appointed time arrived, I entered the interview room nervously. Each member of the panel introduced themselves. I recognised some as leading members of the profession. Other names meant little to me but one I registered was a statistician. Thanks to my advance preparation, things went reasonably smoothly until I was asked about the mathematical validity of using the mathematical Chi Square test for analysing logarithmically derived data. This was foreign territory for me but, rather than expose my ignorance, I explained that I had very recently explored this question with a statistician at the University of London, who was satisfied with its application. The answer was accepted by the panel. I was thanked politely for presenting an intriguing hypothesis and for my time. I returned their thanks and left, feeling reasonably hopeful, and once more called home from a nearby phone box. I noted in passing, the cards on the kiosk wall, offering exotic services that, to my knowledge, were not currently available in Belfast.

A few days later, Mike Dillon phoned me to say he had heard I was to be offered the Fellowship.

tin

Day to day diagnoses

Back in Belfast following those career-defining visits, I became engrossed in dealing with the common problems seen by any children's doctor. I had little time during working hours to dwell on the prospect of more exciting times ahead, working at the national centre of excellence. Problems which might have been considered professionally mundane, yet presented challenges for me beyond merely making a diagnosis, and encouraged the development of the essential skill of alleviating families' anxiety.

Laxatives for diarrhoea

Obesity in children would eventually become a media headline topic but I was sometimes faced with the less-fashionable eating disorders of early childhood. These resulted, for some, in unfortunate upsets in bowel function; in others poor weight gain. Many of the parents I counselled were convinced or terrified that there was some serious underlying disease, which was rarely the case. It took considerable tact to persuade a mother, distressed by her boy's frequent uncontrolled soiling of his pants, that it was not due to bowel cancer, or chronic infective diarrhoea, or some rare food allergy she had read about in the newspaper.

In reality, such an unfortunate symptom was most likely due to chronic constipation and faecal impaction in his lower bowel. Demonstrating this on an abdominal X-ray helped. It was difficult to sell the idea that hardened lumps of faeces, too painful to pass, had blocked the rectum, causing liquid material from higher up the intestines to leak out uncontrollably, thereby relieving the buildup of pressure. I knew a boy in my own primary school who, I realised in retrospect, suffered from this problem, known as encopresis. Sadly, he was known as Stinker Morton. The psychological impact of this was probably lifelong. Treatment is therefore urgent.

Incredulity was a common response whenever I explained that the appropriate treatment was a type of laxative which softened the brick hard faeces.

"Are you seriously suggesting I give my boy laxatives when he already has diarrhoea?"

Offence could be taken if I recommended switching to a healthier, high roughage diet. Mothers do not deliberately feed their children poor diets. I tactfully avoided describing their meals as consisting mainly of rubbish, at least initially. I also had to consider that there might be undisclosed difficulties in a family. On one occasion, I wondered why it was the grandparents who always brought the child along to the clinic. Subsequently, as they came to trust my advice, I learnt it was because the mother was in drug rehab.

In the days before hospital bed numbers were slashed, it was possible to admit a child for a short period and demonstrate to the most unconvinced or sceptical parent that the treatment was effective.

At another clinic, I was told that a small child would eat nothing but cornflakes and milk. I found this almost impossible to believe. My scepticism was unfortunately conveyed by my manner, precipitating tears. I backed off to reconsider. Unsurprisingly, a blood test revealed that the pale faced patient was anaemic and should urgently start iron and vitamin supplements. The supportive input of a clinical psychologist and a helpful dietician was as important as mine.

I saw children whose family doctors had detected a heart murmur, perhaps when carrying out a chest examination during a respiratory infection. A little girl was typical. She was the most active of three siblings, and did not easily get short of breath. Indeed she did not have any symptoms but her doctor reckoned it wise to have any possible underlying heart problem excluded before she came to any harm. My examination revealed a normal Blood Pressure and a regular pulse. It was not unexpected but nevertheless a relief to be only able to detect a soft blowing sound with my stethoscope, confined to one area over her chest when she was lying down, and also because it disappeared as she sat up. Investigations confirmed, as I expected, that there was no underlying structural problem. I was able to explain that her family doctor had simply heard an innocent murmur, caused by normal blood flow through the heart. I was reminded of the panic in my own family many years before when my young sister was referred to hospital for the same reason. There is a special pleasure in seeing a happy family leave the clinic.

I was referred children who frequently woke the family at night with repeated bouts of coughing. Listening to one such a boy's chest revealed a slight wheeze and, by measuring how strongly he could blow into a peak flow meter, I confirmed he had mild asthma. Most of the consultation was taken up with reassurance and explaining how to use an inhaler which should eradicate his symptoms. The boy was more interested in my suggestion that, as a result, he might be able to run faster and be a more successful footballer; a good selling point for the treatment. I recommended that he become a regular swimmer. Sometimes, I involved my patients in challenging parents who smoked to take the same flow meter test, to see whether they could beat their child's result. The children enjoyed this but parents often declined, not realising an adult can generally produce a higher peak flow than any child, given that their lungs are perhaps twice the size. I hoped the message behind the suggestion bore fruit.

The news for families was not always positive. A boy had been taken to see the family doctor because his walking had become ungainly and he was no longer able to keep up with his friends when running. It transpired that he had also developed trouble climbing stairs, only going up one step at a time. While we talked, he sat on the floor playing with some toys. I asked him to bring one over. I noted that he rolled over onto his tummy to get up and held onto a chair to pull himself upright. My heart sank a little as I recognised that he undoubtedly had muscular dystrophy, a condition which would gradually get worse. I wondered if his parents had any inkling of the diagnosis and its implications. I asked if they had any further worries. I then explained I would need to conduct some blood tests and summoned my best efforts to gently introduce the possible diagnosis to them. While a play therapist led the boy off to do some finger painting, I answered their questions as honestly as I could. While the boy was distracted, he allowed a nurse to apply some anaesthetic cream to his arm, so that the necessary diagnostic blood test would be painless. I was able to arrange for a physiotherapy appointment for the following morning and arranged to join

165

the family there with the test results. Shaking their hands as they left, I was thankful that both parents had come along and were able to support each other. A father's attendance at hospital appointments was relatively unusual at that time. Every day I was reminded that small children are parents' most precious possession. I allowed myself a few minutes to reflect and recover from the tension of the appointment before calling the next patient in.

A visit to Hampstead

While patients with a wide spectrum of complaints and illness filled my days, I continued to plan ahead. Armed with the offer of an MRC training fellowship at my annual interview with the postgraduate medical training body, I gained their approval for my proposed career development. They agreed that I should be granted two years unpaid leave of absence from my current post, which would be held open for my return. They had consulted with my employers and this was a calculated decision to ensure I would return, and bring the new expertise I gained back with me. I was pleasantly surprised when the hospital awarded me a travelling scholarship, which I could use to help cover the family's moving expenses. There was now a clear expectation that I would return to develop a dialysis and transplant service for children.

We had three months to get organised for the move to London. Anne gave notice on the nursing post in adult surgery, which she loved. Fortuitously, I heard of a trainee heart surgeon who was transferring from Dublin to gain some further experience in the cardiac surgery unit in Belfast. The timing of his visit matched mine in London. He and his family called to view our home and it was quickly agreed that they would rent it while we were away. We, however, needed to find somewhere affordable to live in London, where rental rates were frighteningly high. Having contacted some rental agencies, and sought advice from a few people we knew there, we booked a few nights in a cheap hotel off Russell Square, near Great Ormond Street as a base to start house hunting. We flew to London full of optimism at what we thought of as the start of a great adventure. Our first stop was a courtesy call at Professor Barratt's office. He confirmed that as a research fellow, I did not qualify for hospital-owned accommodation, but we had a list of properties to view.

The first was just around the corner from the hospital, above an art shop. It was grubby, smelled damp and the toilet was accessed through a tiny kitchen area, which was really an oven and sink on one wall of a short corridor. Our two-year-old son set about happily exploring the premises and we returned to the living room to find he had emptied a pile of pornographic magazines from a cupboard. The agent snatched these from him, as we thanked him and left. It was an unfortunate start.

The next property was nearby on Southampton Row. A private apartment identical to some which the hospital leased, it was perfect, but the cost exceeded my entire monthly research salary. A pattern developed as the day wore on. Anything we could have afforded was so squalid we would not have dreamt of living there, and anything we considered acceptable was outside our price range. After two days we realised we had been naive and needed to search for something much further out, preferably near a tube line which I could use to travel to work. We had no real idea where to look next and had run out of time, as we were booked to travel home the following day.

On the positive side, Mark had enjoyed flying on a plane, eating in restaurants and burger bars, travelling on the underground train, and playing in Coram's Fields, a park near the hospital with a sign at the entrance, "No adults admitted unless accompanied by a child."

Before we packed up, we called in to say goodbye and update the Professor. His secretary, overhearing our tale of woe, started rummaging through a tray of papers. She vaguely remembered some sort of circular that had arrived from The Medical Research Council that afternoon, and which she thought might be helpful.

We all looked at her expectantly.

"Yes, here it is, a major banking group has an apartment they are willing to make available to a suitable medical researcher at a nominal rent," she smiled triumphantly. Anne and I exchanged a hopeful glance.

Martin Barratt took the flyer and read it carefully.

"It's in Hampstead." he said, "and is to be awarded on a first come, first served basis following a satisfactory interview with a senior member of the bank staff, who occupies the main body of the house. There is a phone number here."

He picked up his phone, dialled the number, identified himself, and talked at some length, explaining he had a new research fellow with him who was returning home first thing next day but was anxious to finalise accommodation arrangements. Politely, we tried to pretend we were not hanging on his every word.

He hung up and announced, "they are willing to see you at 7 p.m. this evening. All three of you!"

So, shortly after seven we were seated on an antique chaise lounge in the banker's living room. His wife diffidently offered tea, which we politely declined. As we chatted, they were interested to learn that Anne was a nurse, and about my plans for developing the kidney transplantation programme. There was an awkward moment when the discussion was interrupted by Mark loudly passing a considerable amount of wind. Everyone ignored this impressive explosion which had clearly given our son some pleasure.

The only personal pronoun our future landlords seemed to use was "one" - rather than I, me, you, we or they. We needed to concentrate in order to follow the resulting, rather stilted conversation. Eventually, we were shaking hands to take our leave, unable to assess what sort of impression we had made.

"Well," said our host as we reached the door, "Professor Barratt speaks very highly of you and one looks forward to having you living down below in August. The MRC and the bank will forward a letting agreement to you in due course. Please let them have your address and details."

"Yes indeed, and one hopes you will not mind a little baby sitting for our two little girls as part of the arrangement," added his wife.

At that point, we did not fully appreciate that we had secured a three-bedroom ground floor apartment in one of the most exclusive areas in London. It was two minutes' walk from Hampstead Heath and less than five from a Northern line tube station. We did, however, have a celebratory drink when we had got Mark off to sleep later in the evening.

13. London and Manchester

London days

A double bed mattress balanced precariously on the roof of our small maroon Ford Escort as I drove up Haverstock Hill from Camden to Hampstead. This was undoubtedly a more hazardous trip than the 400 mile journey we had undertaken just a month before, driving down the length of the country from the Stranraer ferry port in Scotland. On that occasion, the car was packed with our most valuable possessions, including our toddler son. After many restless nights in our rented flat, Anne and I realised that if we continued to sleep in the sagging bed that came with it, we would be crippled. Anne spotted a For Sale advertisement in a local newspaper for an "almost new" bed. Inspection, surprisingly, confirmed the description. The mattress was still sealed in the original polythene factory wrapping. With the help of my new friend, Chris, it was now secured to the top of the car with borrowed rope tied to the front and back bumpers, and to the side door handles. We prayed we would not encounter a police car on the way home.

I'd met Chris on our first Sunday in London, when our doorbell rang. Outside stood a smiling, fair-haired young man about my own age. "Hello, I'm your neighbour from the top flat. I thought I'd come and say hello."

"That is really kind of you. Come in, Come in."

"No, that's ok. I really wanted to know if you fancied joining me for a pint in the Coach and Horses?"

I was taken aback.

"But it's Sunday," I spluttered.

"Yes, and it's half past twelve already."

In the 1970s, Northern Irish pubs did not open on Sunday, nor indeed did most shops. In some towns, even children's play parks were closed, with the swings and roundabouts padlocked. It was called The Lord's Day, a day for religious observance only, not for any form of enjoyment.

I could not refuse his offer of friendship and, with Anne's permission, went along to enjoy this aspect of English culture. Forty years later we would join him, his wife Sue and their family and friends, just down the road in

169

another London pub to celebrate his 70th birthday. With good humour, he reminded me of the night we'd walked to the Coach and Horses when a passing motorbike backfired. He watched in puzzlement as I dived behind a parked car. London was a safer place than Belfast, we soon came to realise. Before long, Anne stopped offering puzzled doormen her handbag, expecting them to search it for bombs or guns - a routine requirement in Belfast.

Our first weeks settling in were hectic. Anne explored the local area and located a play group in a nearby Friends Meeting House. This proved a godsend as, although the grand, five-storey town house of which our flat was a part had an extensive rear garden, we had no access to it. The garden was for the sole use of our landlords, who lived in the two main floors. Mark could see their children playing below from our windows and was unable to understand why he could not join them. Soon we made good friends through work, the playgroup and with Chris's wife, Sue, and their daughter Emily, who was Mark's age.

In the university laboratory, I was learning new skills, from simple techniques like using micropipettes, to performing more complex measurements of specific plasma components by using radioactive chemical labels. I was mentored by Vanita Shah, the scientist who worked with Dr Mike Dillon. She proved to be a tolerant teacher, with a great sense of humour, especially when it came to my initial clumsy efforts. She educated me not just in scientific methods and biochemical assay techniques, but also in Asian cuisine. When she discovered I had never eaten pomegranates, lychees and other fruits and vegetables which I considered exotic, she brought me examples to try. Such exotic fruits, chilies, okra, sweet potatoes, and even peppers, which would all have been difficult to find back home.

My research was related to the damage caused to immature kidneys by urine infection. Infection confined to the bladder (cystitis) usually clears quickly with antibiotic treatment. It was known however that when the infection spreads upwards to infect a still developing kidney it could cause residual scarring. One patient in 10 with such damage would in time develop high blood pressure. It was also known that kidneys produce a chemical known as renin or angiotensin in response to reduced renal blood flow. The chemical is powerful at raising the blood pressure in order to keep vital organs perfused, for example after a traumatic blood loss. I suspected that poor blood flow through scarred areas of kidney tissue might simulate that scenario, so that excess renin was produced in some cases. My hypothesis was that this overproduction, in turn, raised the blood pressure unnecessarily.

To test this theory, I set about identifying 100 children with scarred kidneys from the hospital records. I obtained ethical consent to approach their families to take part in my research project. This proved extremely time-consuming. I wished to measure the children's plasma renin activity. I hoped to identify the 10 per cent who might become hypertensive by identifying those with high levels of renin before their blood pressure rose. This would facilitate early intervention to prevent hypertensive complications. Vanita quickly taught me how to measure the renin in the blood samples, using a technique known as radioimmunoassay.

My experience as a clinician was also being expanded, not just in the renal ward to which I was attached, but because the hospital was a national referral centre for difficult or complex patients. Dr Dillon seemed to attract those which were, initially, difficult to even categorise. Unusual cases were often presented by various eminent specialists at weekly teaching sessions. Listening on one occasion, I realised a child I had accompanied to London for investigation some years before was one of the only three cases so far diagnosed in the country of a rare metabolic disorder.

I was gaining exposure to every kidney condition which presents in children. It was pleasing to be immediately accepted as part of the renal team and quickly taught the technique of setting up and managing emergency peritoneal dialysis. At first, when on call for nephrology, I took the precaution of having reference medical texts to hand at home, to consult if necessary. Advice sought by phone from around the country both tested and increased my knowledge and confidence.

I quickly became disenchanted with travelling on the London underground. The carriages were tightly packed with humanity when my train stopped at Hampstead. I needed to almost throw myself through the doors to get on board. I now understood why Professor Barrett and others rode motorbikes. There was little space to park a car at the hospital and I was definitely not entitled to a slot. Soon, I too purchased a second hand 90cc Honda moped and took my life into my own hands amidst the London traffic.

No pressure

Late one evening, I watched as a fax machine regurgitated a page of blood biochemistry results, loaded by a scientist in a distant laboratory. I had been surprised to learn that out of hours at Great Ormond Street Hospital, certain samples were taxied to another hospital for analysis. Back in Belfast we had a 24-hour service on site. I looked at the figures, which were dangerously elevated, and concluded that urgent dialysis was necessary. By phone I consulted with my boss, who concurred.

I walked briskly through the corridors, quiet at that time of night, to the brightly lit cardiac intensive care unit. I was met by the patient's heart surgeon. He listened carefully to my analysis and asked a few pertinent questions in a mid-European accent. He accompanied me to speak briefly with the child's mother. She adjusted her hijab nervously and listened intently to what I had to say. As I described the dialysis process and the essential minor operation involved in setting it up, her brow furrowed and her dark eyes glistened. Choked, she declined to speak, only nodding in acknowledgement several times. She bent over her heavily sedated little boy and whispered softly in his ear, using a language I did not understand. The two-year-old looked pale and fragile, the scar and stitches from his recent surgery hidden by a patterned blue sheet. Attached to his chest and arms were the sensors of various monitors. His mother kissed his forehead, turned to nod to me again with her palms pressed together, offered her thanks, and left the cubicle with one of the nursing staff.

Shortly, another nurse arrived with a sterile peritoneal dialysis pack and we introduced ourselves. She informed me she had assisted with this procedure several times and, as I scrubbed up, she set up a drip stand. I chose an appropriate dialysis fluid, she checked its temperature, hung it on the stand, and then ran some through the heated tubing of the delivery system.

We talked over the operation plan step by step. The pack was opened and checked, and nurse Stevens poured antiseptic Savlon solution, surgical spirit, and iodine into three little plastic pots.

172

"Thanks, it's great that setting up dialysis isn't new to you, you'll be able to keep me right," I said with a grin. "I'll do my best, but please call me Marcia," she replied, also smiling.

After we had both scrubbed up and donned sterile gowns and gloves, I cleaned the skin over the child's lower abdomen with each fluid in turn. He was sedated and had a low dose morphine infusion running, and so did not stir. I asked Marcia to break open a vial of local anaesthetic. She held it up first so that I could read the label, saying, "Lignocaine, one percent".

I read it and agreed, "Lignocaine, one percent".

I relaxed a little, appreciating that she was both friendly and efficient. I chose a midline spot for the incision, one third of the way between the umbilicus and the upper edge of the pelvic pubic bone. This is below where the major midline vessels, the arterial aorta and the vena cava, divide and branch towards the upper legs. Penetrating the abdomen there, safely avoids these vital structures. I injected the lignocaine into the skin and muscle fascia of the abdominal wall. We waited for it to take effect.

"Are you from Ireland? I haven't seen you around before?"

For the first time I noticed her accent.

"Yes, I'm from Belfast. I've only been working here for a couple of months. And you?"

"An Aussie, working and travelling for a couple of years up north."

She handed the dialysis line to me, the tubing now filled with fluid. I attached an intravenous needle and cannula to the end, tested that the patient's skin was numb, then advanced it carefully through the abdominal wall. Once the needle point entered the abdominal cavity, the fluid ran in rapidly, which allows the loops of bowel to float safely out of the way. I removed the sharp ended needle, leaving the plastic cannula in place, and infused more fluid through it.

Now came the moment that required total concentration.

First, I removed the cannula, then made a tiny incision with a scalpel. The nurse opened out a packet containing a larger plastic dialysis catheter which had a metal stylet inside the hollow lumen with its extremely sharp point protruding beyond the end. The stylet resembled a rather dangerously honed knitting needle. I needed to pass this through the abdominal wall, avoiding any underlying organs, aiming it behind the bladder so it could pass deep into the pelvic cavity, below and away from any large blood vessels. I took a deep breath. It required considerable but controlled pressure to push the instrument through the tissues without the spike penetrating too deeply. Marcia attempted to relieve the tension of the moment.

"Have you heard the story going around, that this little one may actually be some sort of prince?" she remarked, conversationally.

At that moment, thankfully, I felt a pop and the fluid we had infused welled up along the catheter tube. I knew I'd safely penetrated the peritoneal cavity and quickly withdrew the metal stylet, while advancing the soft plastic catheter deeper into position. The fluid began to drain into a sterile bag. It was slightly yellow but transparent, There was no blood staining. We could relax.

I secured the tube in place with a stitch and Marcia taped it down, I pulled off my face mask.

"I have to say your timing in letting me know that I might be stabbing royalty was perfect." I remarked, grinning with relief. "You nearly gave me a heart attack just then."

Marcia put a hand over her mouth. "Oh! Ooh! Sorry!"

"That's okay," I told her, "I have to confess that I don't set up dialysis often in the middle of the night, so thank you, I think we made a good team."

I never did learn whether our patient was an actual Prince. To me, he was just a sick little boy.

Peritoneal dialysis is efficient in correcting deranged biochemistry in small children, when the kidney purification filter fails. It is a relatively simple process. The scientifically designed fluid contains dextrose and electrolytes. A volume, determined by the patient's size, is run into the abdomen, left for a time, then drained out. With each cycle, waste products and chemicals pass into the fluid and are removed, in this instance lowering a critically high level of potassium, which can cause a disordered heart rhythm and even a cardiac arrest. We used fluid containing no dissolved potassium. The high level of potassium in the blood flowing through the vessels in the peritoneum therefore moves spontaneously by osmosis into the dialysis fluid and is removed.

Our patient's heart operation was a success and the period of dialysis bought time for his kidneys to gradually recover from the insult to them caused by being under-perfused with blood at the time of the open heart surgery, during which his circulation was maintained by a mechanical pump, bypassing the heart.

While my nervousness settled within minutes, his kidneys took several days to recover.

Einstein is not so clever

My research was beginning to produce encouraging results. The positive response to my letters seeking participants in the study was a tribute to the high esteem in which the hospital staff were held by the families of children they looked after. I enjoyed the challenges of the work and developed several side projects - but there was still no long-term chronic renal replacement programme in the hospital. In order to gain experience in haemodialysis and transplantation I needed to move elsewhere at the end of my year. A post at Guy's Hospital, near London Bridge, would have been ideal, as many Great Ormond Street patients were referred there for further treatment. I applied and was shortlisted for the job but, disappointingly, it was awarded to an in-house candidate.

Professor Barratt recommended I apply to The Albert Einstein Hospital in New York, a leading international centre in our field. An international fellowship in nephrology had become available there - and in December of 1977 I learned that my application was successful. One hurdle remained. I needed written confirmation of employment before the new year in order to obtain a work visa. I held the education certificate for foreign medical graduates which qualified me to work in the United States. However, a new visa qualifying examination would be required for applications filed after 1 January. There would be no opportunity to sit this test before the change took effect. I made this clear to the hospital and my mentor in the States, Professor Spitzer. He confirmed that the required documentation would reach me shortly. As Christmas approached, I made several anxious transatlantic phone calls and received reassurances each time that the papers had been posted. I was at first frustrated, then extremely disappointed, when they eventually arrived too late, in early January.

Incredibly, they had been sent by surface rather than air mail. Professor Spitzer, embarrassed by the clerical mistake, attempted to have the regulations waived, and I even accompanied him to the American Embassy in London on his next visit to Europe. He presented a letter from the state department office, supporting the granting of an exemption. It had no effect.

I remained stoical and worked on as before. After presenting preliminary results of my research at a national forum, I was approached by the paediatric nephrology team in Manchester. They could offer all the experience I required. After a short interview, I was offered a clinical lectureship, starting in the autumn.

Meanwhile, it was fascinating to work in a national centre, where I encountered high profile visitors including Queen Elizabeth II and the world boxing champion Mohammed Ali. Mohammed was the children's favourite. He arrived with an enormous cake and several pairs of boxing gloves. Mock sparring with the ill girls and boys and pretending to be knocked out allowed them to forget how sick they were. We didn't get such exciting visits in Belfast.

Decisions

I was by now experienced in counselling parents facing difficult decisions, sometimes life and death decisions. I tried to picture myself in their position. When we talked, I endeavoured to use language and detail they could understand as they weighed up treatment options. While ready to express my preferred course of action, if asked, I was careful not to prejudge their conclusions. I always attempted to give them hope, if possible.

On one occasion, Anne and I were faced with a difficult decision to make ourselves.

As summer arrived, we arranged a holiday with my brother, his wife, and two nieces in Devon. Some weeks before we were due to leave, Anne told me she thought she was pregnant. We were delighted but I reflected that, perhaps, it was fortunate we were not after all going to America. It was only then that we realised we had not registered with a local family doctor.

Anne now did so and arranged an appointment, primarily to have the pregnancy confirmed. She entered the doctor's consulting room and was invited to sit down.

"I understand you have moved here recently from Ireland and believe you may be pregnant," he suggested.

Anne confirmed this, and began to explain we had moved to London some time ago, but had not needed a doctor - partly because she was a nurse, and I was medically qualified. Before she could make this clear, he interrupted.

"So, you are interested in arranging an abortion?"

Abortion was illegal throughout Ireland, but not in England. He assumed this was why we'd come over to the UK.

Anne was stunned and appalled by his crass attitude and prejudiced conclusion, which he'd reached without listening. She was still boiling with rage when I returned home in the evening and heard the story. I shared her disgust.

This did not spoil the news when the pregnancy test proved positive.

Soon, we were in Devon and enjoying the sunshine and sea air with my brother and his family. On the second day, as the children were changing into swimwear on the beach, our nieces appeared to have developed a pink skin rash. I was called upon to suggest a diagnosis. I examined the rash and detected little glands behind their ears and concluded they probably had German measles - rubella. We were forced to reveal our secret news, then hastily set off to find a public phone so we could ask Anne's mother if she had contracted rubella as a child. Her mum couldn't remember for sure. One of her daughters had caught the infection 20 years earlier, but maybe it was both?

We packed a few essentials and drove 200 miles back to my laboratory in London. On the same floor, my friend Bill Marshall, an infectious disease specialist, also had an office. He immediately agreed to take a blood sample to check Anne for rubella antibodies, which would be proof of past infection. We had a long overnight wait for the result. We ate at a local restaurant, barely interested in the food as we discussed the potential risk to our unborn baby, and what we might do if Anne didn't have the protective antibodies.

177

Worried and uncertain, we agreed not to make a decision until we knew the blood result, and returned to our flat as darkness fell.

A police raid

We turned on the television, made some coffee and settled down to try and watch the day's events at the Wimbledon Tennis Championships. Suddenly, we were alarmed by loud hammering at the front door and the insistent ringing of the bell ringing, We switched on the entrance hall and outside lights and opened the door. A very large policeman stood there, another could be seen in the blue flashing lights from their car.

"You live here, don't you?" He asked. "May I come in?"

We retreated back to the living room, and asked, "What exactly is going on?"

"Your landlord upstairs called in to say the tenants in their ground floor apartment were away on holiday and they believed they could hear noises below. He suspected there might be burglars inside."

Already in an anxious state, we responded with a few uncomplimentary words about our neighbours, pointing out that our car could easily be seen parked outside. The constable offered a suggestion.

"Maybe you should use your phone and let him know you are home."

We briefly explained our situation to the understanding police officer. I omitted the personal details of why we had returned and made a tactfully apologetic call to our haughty landlord.

With the police gone and the neighbours placated, we retired to bed and attempted to sleep.

Early the next day, Dr Marshall delivered good news. Anne was immune. The baby was safe.

We hit the road back to Devon to share the good news and restart our holiday.

The next year flew by, and we made lifelong friends. I worked alongside and learned from colleagues from all corners of the world, from Finland to Greece, from Asia and Australia to America. Klaus from Hanover, a partner in some of the hypertension studies, became our fallback babysitter.

His excellent spoken English was not, however, fully appreciated by our son. He complained to us that Klaus couldn't do the proper voices for his favourite bedtime stories.

Moving on, I would miss the laboratory work with Vanita, the team scientist, and the regular advice of my clinical and research mentors, with whom I was now on first name terms. Pretension was foreign to Mike and Martin's nature, despite their world class status in science, nephrology and paediatrics. I recognised in them an ability to focus on the most difficult clinical problems with a sharp intellect, passion and compassion, which I would try to emulate. We shared a vision of finding successful treatments for kidney diseases in children. They were determined to understand the mechanisms behind these conditions. They tempted me to stay and pursue a career in scientific research and academia. However, my thoughts inevitably returned to the children back home, who had no access to renal dialysis or transplantation. I had concentrated on this as my primary mission for several years.

On one of my last weekends on call, Mark, then aged three, decided to come with me to the ward for the Sunday morning handover meeting. He sat quietly in the corner, enjoying some juice and a biscuit as this progressed. I described a child who had come in from Kings Lynn overnight, detailing their signs, symptoms, blood results and the treatment I had initiated.

"I think that's the whole story, as I understand it. I don't think I have left anything out." There was a pause as the team weighed up the information. In the silence, a child's voice piped up, "You haven't told them the blood pressure."

Dr Dillon looked at Mark with a broad smile. "You are quite right, young man," he said and gazed back at me questioningly.

"Actually, it was normal," I reported.

"It seems your young assistant has grasped the importance of the blood pressure in kidney disease. It's lucky you brought him along."

Mark continued munching a biscuit.

A farewell dinner

One of the other senior academics on our floor generously hosted a dinner party, inviting the year's research fellows and their partners to his home. His wife had arranged the seating so that partners were separated. I found myself sitting next to the hostess. I congratulated her on the tender chicken and delicious sauce.

"Yes, thank you, the jus is my own secret recipe," she informed me, "but actually, the meat is veal." I apologised and wondered how I might salvage the conversation. She helped me.

"Your wife? What has she been doing in London?"

"Anne is a surgical nurse normally, but with a toddler to look after here, with no family back up and a constant stream of visitors, she has taken a career break. She enjoys helping at a play group and has made quite a few friends." I sipped some wine and added," May I ask, apart from being an excellent cook, do you work?"

"I teach."

"At which level? Primary or secondary school?"

The reply was short.

"Royal College of Music. Cello."

At this, she rose to suggest the men move on two seats clockwise around the table, before a sweet course was served. I was very happy to escape, feeling I may have revealed a certain lack of sophistication. Anne savoured my report of the conversation on the way home.

I had, by now, gained a broad knowledge of the range of kidney diseases of childhood, become competent in their diagnosis and management, and in delivering acute peritoneal dialysis. I had presented three research papers at nephrology conferences and spent my last month refining these for submission and for eventual publication in scientific medical journals.

I sold my trusty motorbike to a new research fellow and would not regret running the gauntlet of the dense London traffic or breathing the fumes it produced. Our car was once again packed full. Travelling ahead of us, in a large van, were several packing cases, crammed with items we had

180

accumulated in London (including a child-sized, pedal-driven police car, a present from Mark's grandmother).

On our final morning, our landlord called to say goodbye and wish us well, but also to check for breakages. He then departed in his chauffeur-driven limousine for the city, wearing his uniform: Bowler hat, pinstripe suit, long dark coat with velvet collar, and a briefcase.

It had been a special year, but we looked forward to new challenges and, of course, a new baby.

Manchester

"Ta-rah, luv," called the lady in the corner shop. "Ta-rah," My son called back waving goodbye with an ice lolly. It was a Saturday morning ritual to spend an hour in the nearby play park, and to buy a treat and the newspaper on the way home.

The locals here were friendly by nature. They offered a "hello" as they passed in the street. The corner shop lady knew exactly who all her customers were. Other children lived in our street and it was safe for buddies to run between each other's houses. Mark loved the nearby Lake's Nursery School, where he claimed his favourite teacher was called Mrs. Astursika. Was he mispronouncing this? No, it transpired that this was indeed her name - and she was as kindly as he reported.

When we moved north, The Royal Manchester Hospital allocated us a second floor maisonette in Swinton, a few miles away from the site. It seemed perfect accommodation at first, until we grew to detest the constant noise from the adjacent motorway traffic on opening any window. Most of our neighbours were elderly and a little intolerant of a small, noisy boy. There was no elevator and hauling a buggy, shopping and a toddler up two flights of stairs was quite an effort for a pregnant mum. The decor, furniture, fittings, utensils and equipment were all brand new, so we hesitated to complain. Mark had no outside play space or nearby playmates there. Then he developed mumps and an associated viral meningitis. We had had enough of Swinton, and managed to relocate to a house that backed onto the hospital grounds and had several junior doctors living on either side. The house was less than pristine. The floors and carpets were extremely grubby and the oven was filthy, with a skillet stuck in congealed grease on a tray inside. There was a pervading musty smell, identifiable as stale curry. A major clean-up was required. We purchased a second hand Keymatic washing machine which had four programmes, depending on which side of the square plastic control key was inserted. It developed a social circle of its own, as none of the adjacent hospital houses boasted any such domestic appliances. We embarked on a deep clean programme, shampooing carpets and removing grime from kitchen appliances, walls surfaces. This included washing the curtains and loose furnishings in the trusty machine. There was considerable shrinkage in some material and the front room curtains subsequently failed to reach the windowsills. Later, we discovered this discrepancy gave our neighbours an advantage when they wanted to do some laundry, as they could always tell if we were at home and awake.

In the hospital, I concentrated on clinical work rather than research. The two paediatric nephrologists proved to be a pleasure to work with. Ian Houston, the professor of paediatrics, made me extremely welcome. Bob Postlethwaite was a year younger than me but already held a consultant post. He and I developed a special and fruitful working relationship.

The Professor proposed that, initially, the alternate night and weekend rota should continue unaltered, with me shadowing him when he was on call so that I could learn the ropes. Before long, I became more competent under his tutelage and the rota shifted so that he was rarely called upon after dark. This suited my desire for practical experience - and he made no objection.

Operating in the dark

Glomerulonephritis is an inflammatory kidney condition of variable severity. Frequently, tissue is required for microscopic analysis in order to make a definitive diagnosis, classify the pathology, predict the outcome, and design treatment. In order to avoid a major operation involving exposing the kidney and directly dissecting out a small sample, a technique was developed that allowed us to use a biopsy needle to extract a small core of renal tissue. Bob was skilled at this and set about teaching me how to successfully pass the needle through the skin and into a patient's kidney. Initially I watched, then assisted him. Next, he assisted me, until he was satisfied I was competent to carry out the procedure safely and unsupervised.

The first time I did so, Bob retired to his nearby office. I was assisted only by a nurse, who monitored the prone patient and ensured he remained still. During the procedure, she sat at the boy's head, monitoring his breathing and resting one hand on each shoulder. The patient had first been heavily sedated in the ward, then moved to the adjacent radiology department once he was asleep. With the child lying on his tummy, the area on his back over the kidney was frozen with local anaesthetic and the skin sterilised with various antiseptics. I injected some opaque liquid radio contrast medium into a vein in the arm. I could control the X-ray image intensifier using a foot pedal to switch the radiation briefly on and off. The lights were dimmed so that I could more easily see the dye accumulate in and outline the kidney on the screen. I selected a fine guide needle and passed it down into the delineated lower third. As the sleeping child breathed in and out, the kidney moved up and down, as now did the fine probe needle. This confirmed it was in the correct position. Once in place, I noted the depth of the kidney below the skin. I withdrew the needle and made a tiny incision with a scalpel. I picked up the considerably larger biopsy needle, which was slightly narrower in diameter than a writing pencil. I pushed it gently through the little incision, following the probe's track.

An enormous crash echoed through the gloom of the radiology theatre.

I had already advanced the needle near to the kidney surface but was forced to let go and look around. The nurse had collapsed to the floor in a faint.

Once the needle is in the kidney, it must only be held during the natural pause between breathing in and breathing out, when the organ does not move. To keep holding on while the patient breathes, will cause the needle to tear through the mobile soft kidney tissue as the organ moves. This may cause an internal haemorrhage.

I rapidly assessed the situation and decided to ignore the nurse and quickly, and safely, completed the biopsy and withdrew the needle. I then phoned for assistance, as the nurse started to struggle to her feet. I instructed her to stay lying down as I checked on the patient who happily remained asleep, oblivious to the drama.

Within 20 minutes, both child and nurse were fully recovered and under the expert care of the unflappable ward sister. I retired to have a much-needed cup of tea and discuss the events with my colleague. The biopsy report from the pathologist showed a form of glomerulonephritis with a low likelihood of progression.

I never again fully relaxed while carrying out these biopsies, until, learning from this event, I was able to perform them in an operating theatre with the patient under a full anaesthetic controlled by an anaesthetist, assisted by a surgical scrub nurse and with a radiographer operating the scanner.

As the months passed, Anne's pregnancy advanced smoothly, marred only by an unpleasant encounter with an obstetrician recommended by a friend and colleague in Belfast who had looked after Anne before Mark was born. Sadly, his colleague in England had none of George's kindness, warmth, or humour. He managed with inappropriate rudeness during her first straightforward consultation, to reduce my happy, level-headed wife to tears. I wondered how young women without Anne's character and nursing experience coped with his brusque arrogance. Fortunately, none of his pompous personality rubbed off on the midwives.

A sad visit home

Towards Christmas I answered a call from my brother, who said I should make a trip home immediately, or I might not have the opportunity to see my father alive again. This was the man who had inspired my love of children and who, despite having no academic background, had encouraged his own children to attend college and university. He and my mother had at times taken on one or more extra part-time jobs to ensure this was possible. He had gradually recovered from his first stroke a few years earlier - but on the day, a year later, that he returned to his job, he suffered the first of several more. He was now unconscious in hospital, my mother having finally admitted that she and my sister could no longer nurse him at home. I immediately made travel arrangements, although I worried about leaving Anne behind with only a couple of months before her due date.

It was indeed the last time I saw my father alive. He seemed completely unaware of his surroundings as I sat alone next to his bed. I thanked him for all he had done for me. I told him I was carrying on the work he did with children. His had been a spiritual calling, mine merely medical. I sat and held his hand. I doubted that much of what I was trying to say reached him. I told him I loved him, which he undoubtedly knew. After an overnight visit, I sadly kissed him and my mother goodbye, and returned to my family and my work.

Haemodialysis

In the Royal Manchester Children's Hospital at Pendlebury, there was no haemodialysis provision. That was located instead at a facility located some miles away at the Booth Hall Children's Hospital. Our team travelled there once or twice a week to review each patient. In this type of treatment, the patient's blood is diverted from a large forearm vessel and passed through a machine, which pumps it through an artificial kidney before returning it to normal circulation. Inside this device, blood passes along one side of an artificial semipermeable membrane and a dialysis solution flows in the opposite direction along the other side. This countercurrent system maximises the removal of toxic solutes from the blood. The machines are expensive and require a specially-treated water supply to produce the dialysis solution. This solution draws only waste products, excess water and chemicals such as potassium across the membrane which separates it from direct contact with the blood. The type of membrane, the pressure exerted across the membrane, and the composition of the solution is tailored to each individual patient to achieve the optimum correction of their blood chemistry. I needed to be proficient in managing haemodialysis if I was to initiate a similar programme in Belfast.

As I observed and learnt this technique, my interest was also drawn to an alternative; a type of peritoneal dialysis (PD) which had the potential to be employed long term. I thought this might be the first method to introduce when developing a service at home in Belfast. It was relatively low tech. No special facilities were required, beyond those found in any hospital ward - no technicians, no water treatment plant, and it was highly efficient in small children. It required a catheter to be inserted semi-permanently in the abdominal (peritoneal) cavity. The material used was soft and rested relatively comfortably against the skin, and the catheter had attached Teflon cuffs, which sealed the surgical opening in the peritoneal membrane and the skin as the tissues healed. These catheters could be left in place for many months, or even years. The technique involved a bag of dialysis fluid, of predetermined chemical composition, being attached and run into the abdomen. The fluid was left for several hours to allow waste material and excess fluid to cross the natural peritoneal membrane, which lines the abdominal cavity, and so correct the blood chemistry. The fluid was drained back out into the bag and discarded. Each bag was replaced by a fresh volume of fluid several times during the day. This was a refinement of the technique I had used in London to provide short term dialysis in the cardiac unit. A meticulous, clean technique is essential when attaching and disconnecting successive bags of fluid. If parents could be trained to undertake this treatment in their own home, time spent in hospital would be minimised, as would disruption to a child's schooling and daily life. This process was called chronic ambulatory peritoneal dialysis (CAPD).

In the ward at Pendlebury we were also using an early automated PD machine which repeatedly cycled small volumes of fluid in and out overnight, from its large reservoir. Children could sleep during this process and needed no dialysis during the day. Eventually, we hoped these machines would be refined to become reliable enough for home treatment.

Manchester United calls

On Christmas week, the famous Manchester United football team visited the hospital. They chatted with children and parents and flirted with the nurses. They had footballs and teddy bears in the team colours, red and white. Every boy received a football as a present, the girls and toddlers got a teddy. In the middle of the excitement, I noticed one unhappy boy. He had a rare condition called cystinosis which interferes with both normal growth and kidney function. He was very small for his nine years. As the squad headed for the door, I noticed a discarded bear on the floor beside his bed, and realised what had happened. I caught the last couple of footballers as they were about to leave for the next ward, and explained. They quickly grabbed a ball and dribbled it between them, moving back along the ward. As they reached

Tommy's bed one flicked the ball in the air towards the other, who headed it onto the bed. They chatted with Tommy as they signed the ball and shook hands with him before waving goodbye to everyone.

A death and a birth

While my hospital work held exciting prospects for the future, more importantly and immediately, as the new year dawned, we eagerly anticipated the arrival of our second child.

Then the phone call we had been dreading came. My father had passed away.

Anne's estimated delivery date was only 10 days away. Her parent's response was speedy. Her dad, Joe, flew in from Ireland. He was an old soldier and set about developing a plan. I drove him to the maternity unit,several miles from our house. He drove the car on the return leg of the dummy run so that he was familiar with the route. He was calm and in control as I left for the airport and the funeral in Belfast.

With my mother, I stood at my father's coffin in an upstairs bedroom of our family home. I was anxious not to upset her but failed to stop tears from flowing.

"You are the first one to cry," she whispered, putting her arm around my waist.

My brothers and sister had done a better job of controlling their emotions and hiding their grief when she was present, to avoid her further upset. Far off in England, I had been spared the harrowing months of his final illness.

Our house, garden, and the pavement outside were crowded for the simple Christian service, held in the front room. My father was a man of stalwart faith, gone now to a higher place, free from the undeserved indignity of his suffering. The cortège walked slowly down the road, bringing traffic to a standstill. After the coffin was carried on the shoulders of mourners for half a mile, we placed it in a hearse. As I looked back up the hill, the road was filled as far as the eye could see, with people who had come to pay their respects.The interment and the evening became an emotional blur. I spent a restless night in my old bed and, too soon, it was time to go, yet it was also too long to have been away.

Almost 20 years later, I sat with my mother in her apartment in a fold for elderly people. We were sharing a pot of tea, a Thursday ritual, after we had done her weekly shop. I was telling her some story about one of our children.

"I just wish your father could have been here to enjoy his grandchildren. He was taken too soon."

She had recently had a triple coronary artery bypass herself, at the age of 80.

"It always seemed so unfair for a man who never smoked or drank alcohol, and who walked or cycled everywhere, to die so young."

I agreed, and she continued.

"It was those bombs that destroyed his grocery store which caused his stroke," she said with certainty.

"The first time they struck, he carried the deadly package out to the waste ground beside the shop. I told him never to do anything so foolish again."

I nodded. "I know, but he believed he was known and respected by customers on both sides of the community."

She continued. "He walked to and from work through the republican Ardoyne, and the loyalist Woodvale area next to it without anyone bothering him. He thought he was safe. The shop served both sides, after all.

Then, that terrible afternoon, they came back. Hard men with balaclavas and guns. They cleared every penny from the tills. The bomb was carried to the very back of the shop.

"This time, you have two minutes to get out," they shouted as they ran to the getaway car. Even then, your dad grabbed a bottle of tomato sauce as he fled with the customers and staff. He threw it after the disappearing car. The bomb explosion turned the shop to rubble and his livelihood was wiped out."

She paused and sipped her tea.

"He was never the same again."

On arriving back in Manchester, my father-in-law confided that he doubted he really could remember the route to the hospital. Anne was unconcerned.

188

"Don't worry, dad, I would have kept you right."

A week later I dropped her off there. The midwives promised to phone me if labour began. Early in the morning, Anne began to feel a few contractions. Having heard nothing by 11 o'clock, I phoned in. I was stunned to be told that if I didn't get there at once, I might miss the birth. I raced through the city traffic, abandoned the car, and hurried to the delivery suite. Anne calmed me down, telling me she had just had a shot of pethidine for pain relief. A large, smiling midwife of West Indian extraction breezed in, carried out an examination and confirmed that the cervix was fully dilated. The contractions became stronger.

I was redundant, but Anne seemed to be in control.

"I really need to push down now!" she announced.

"Try lying on your side, love," the nurse suggested, "put your right foot in my armpit and let us see what is happening."

This was a strange new approach to me, but I said nothing.

Anne pushed, breathed hard and pushed again several times.

Shortly she was holding our daughter, Emily, in her arms, named for her great grandmother.

A few months later my mother came to visit. Special time spent with baby Emily helped her through those sad days. I remembered this 18 years later, when I saw my daughter's nickname in her school leaving yearbook, "Little Miss Sunshine".

Organ transplants

I was becoming proficient in managing various forms of dialysis and in performing the procedures and preliminary tests in the workup required before patients were placed on call for a kidney. Each one had their tissue type determined and listed with the UK transplant service. The tissue type is based on their human leucocyte antigen (HLA) profile. The immune system uses the HLA profile to decide which cells belong to a person and which do not. The HLA tissue type of the kidney donor is also analysed and matched by the national computer system to a potential recipient with the same, or very similar, type. This is more complex, but not a lot different to the concept of matching donor and patient blood groups before a transfusion. I attended the weekly kidney transplant meeting at Manchester Royal Infirmary, where all adult and paediatric transplants were carried out. Each patient's tissue type and acceptable level of match or mismatch would be discussed. Tissue matches are rarely perfect, except between identical twins. The body's immune system has the job of attacking viruses and bacteria to fight infection but will also attack any foreign protein or cells it encounters, including that of transplanted organs if the HLA types are poorly matched. A major consideration is always the degree of mismatch between donor and recipient which is considered safe. After an organ transplant, immunosuppressive drugs are used to block the system from attacking and rejecting the patient's new kidney.

Seeing a child who had previously scraped by on dialysis, pale and small for their age, attend a transplant follow-up clinic a few months after surgery in robust health - and now perhaps a little overweight due to immunosuppressive steroid treatment - was a special pleasure.

Pertussis

Family life produced its own rewards and challenges. A neighbour called to ask if we had noticed her little boy, who was frequently in our house, had a bad cough. She wanted us to know that he had been diagnosed by the family doctor as having whooping cough.   Around this time there was a controversial claim, subsequently proven to be unfounded, that pertussis vaccine might rarely cause brain damage.This resulted in as little as one third of children being vaccinated. Emily was three months old. Mark started to cough, and it steadily got worse. It came in staccato bursts, and he was unable to stop until he vomited or his lips turned blue. Only then could he draw in a great breath with the characteristic 'whooping 'noise. We gave Emily regular preventative doses of the antibiotic erythromycin. She may have been under six pounds at birth but proved to be a toughie and escaped the infection.

Throughout all this, Anne continued to donate surplus breast milk to the premature baby unit. It was used not only to feed the tiny patients, but also to treat those with conjunctivitis - an apparently effective remedy due to the natural antibiotics it contains. All part of belonging to the hospital family.

Moratorium

When had lived in Manchester for almost a year, a post was advertised in the British Medical Journal for a paediatrician with a special interest in Nephrology. The appointment was at the Royal Belfast Hospital for Sick Children. I immediately applied and shortly received a date for candidate interviews. On learning I was the only applicant, I gave notice to leave my position in Manchester. We hoped to be back in Belfast in time for Mark to start primary school in September. I would be sorry to be leaving the place in which I had probably enjoyed working the most, so far, in my career.

One afternoon in July, I was attending a case conference about a child with injuries consistent with physical abuse and neglect. A secretary knocked and slipped in to deliver a message. Professor Carré in Belfast was on the phone.I asked her to tell him I would call him back immediately after the meeting finished.

A minute later, she returned to say that Professor Carré had asked her to emphasise that he needed to speak to me urgently, on a matter of some importance. Reluctantly, I gave my apologies to the meeting, and hurried to the nearby office.

"Maurice, I apologise for interrupting you, but I have unfortunate news which you needed to know at once. I'm afraid I have just heard that there has been a moratorium announced on all new NHS consultant posts here, due to budget deficits. The decision was made at the Department of Health this morning."

I was shocked.

"Does this mean the nephrology post and interviews next week will not go ahead?"

"I'm afraid so. I checked once I heard the news. I know you were planning to resign in Manchester and thought I should warn you immediately against doing so."

I sat considering what to do. Mark was almost five years old and had a place to start school in Belfast that autumn. The case conference proceeded without me.

I called the human resources office at the University and explained I wished to withdraw my resignation. I was informed it was too late to do so, as my current post has already been advertised. Thinking quickly, I explained my situation and asked to have an application form sent to me. Worse news followed. The closing date for applications had passed.

The job I had worked towards for years had evaporated.

The Interview

"New suit?" asks the person at the adjacent urinal. Already with a nervous bladder, I am slightly rattled by the English-accented voice, which I do not recognise. I glance sideways, careful to keep my eyes above shoulder height. It is an eminent London renal physician. He recognises me from various research meetings which he chaired, and where I have presented my work. It has been almost a year since I have returned to Belfast from Manchester.

"Actually yes," I replied, looking steadily ahead.

"There are only two occasions when purchasing a new suit is warranted. One for your first consultant interview and the second for your first wedding," he says to the wall.

We turn and wash our hands. He wishes me good luck as we enter the foyer of the university administration building. The funding for the nephrology post has been released after a year's delay, and it is interview day for the applicants. My washroom colleague is the external assessor from the Royal College of Physicians.

Shortly before I was due to return to Belfast, destined for only a senior registrar post, a paediatrician in a local hospital had, conveniently for me but unfortunately for her, tripped over a sign warning of a wet floor. Falling heavily, she suffered a nasty hip fracture. I have been acting as her replacement for the last nine months.

My name is called. I am to be interrogated by eight people, mostly university academics or senior medical consultants. First, my experience and credentials are checked. The chairman then defers to the visiting expert.

"If we were to wheel a haemodialysis machine into the room and we had a patient here, would you be happy to set up for a treatment session?"

"Yes, of course," I reply, describing the procedure in what I hope is a confident voice.

192

Another part of my brain has the ridiculous thought that the door might swing open and a machine wheeled through, but the room only just had space for the large oak table and my inquisitors. They include university and NHS representatives, alongside a city counsellor as a lay representative from the local health committee.

I hastily add, "Although in practice, specialist renal nurses usually perform this task. My role is to supervise and calculate a suitable treatment prescription."

The senior hospital manager wants to know an estimate of the cost of setting up a renal replacement service for children. I give a ballpark figure I have calculated in preparation for such a question. He looks pensive.

Eventually after about an hour, it is the Professor of Greek's turn.

"I have done a little homework and came across two diseases known as nephrotic syndrome and nephritic syndrome. I believe the terms are derived from an old Greek linguistic root. Can you expand?".

"I'm afraid my only real knowledge of ancient Greek is some myths and the Hippocratic Oath," I reply. I groan inwardly. What am I saying? He smiles benignly. I give a brief explanation of the difference in the two conditions. He is pleased with his erudite question, but I doubt if he is really interested in the detailed response.

Suddenly my ordeal is over. The City counsellor rises to open the door.

"Good luck son," he whispers. "I think you've done ok." I nod my thanks for his kindness.

A few days later, I found the panel had agreed with his conclusion. I received a letter of appointment as a senior lecturer in the university, and as a consultant paediatrician with a special interest in nephrology.

14. Consultant nephrologist

We had conflicting emotions when we left Manchester. We knew we would miss our good friends there, and that I would miss the hospital team and the children I had come to know. There were families with whom I had forged a close bond, which would inevitably be lost. A great working relationship with senior colleagues was to morph into lifelong friendship. We were, however, looking forward to getting home to our families and old friends. A parting memento was a print by LS Lowry; one of his famous "pictures of match-stick men" in the industrial northwest of England.

So, I returned as a consultant to the hospital where I first studied childhood diseases as a student, and where I had met Becky, the little girl who could not speak. I remembered her uninhibited greeting on that first day. I wondered if I would somehow be able to encourage the same resilience, warmth and self confidence in the ill children I would look after in my new post. Always at the back of my mind was another little girl, Rachel with inexorably progressive kidney disease, whose illness and prognosis was the impetus for my travel to train in England.

The unit hadn't changed in the 10 years since. There were over 30 cots and beds, three side wards, where patients who required isolation could be cared for, and a nursery annexe for babies and infants. The main area of the old Victorian ward remained divided into three sections by wood partitions of about two metres in height. The upper halves of these were constructed of a transparent plastic, so that the 20 or so patients could be more easily observed by staff. It had an arched, painted, solid plaster ceiling at least four or five metres high, so that every noise bounced around the room. The walls were decorated with watercolour depictions of nursery rhymes, daubed onto glazed tiles. The children in these pictures were dressed in clothes from a bygone age. Eventually, this artwork became the subject of a preservation order. The rest of the walls were a dull beige and green - perhaps befitting, in someone's mind, a hospital. Or maybe it was subconsciously their idea of the colour of sickness.

The ward sister was efficient, if a little spiky, and did not suffer fools gladly. I found her sympathetic to me and my new ideas, not least because we had spent some of our early education at the same primary school in the north of the city.

Gradually, children with every sort of kidney problem were referred to the new service. Early on, I inherited from the surgical team a group of patients with urological problems. They had been following some of them up since birth, or soon after. Urology is the treatment of structural disorders of the urinary system. This consists of the ureters, the tubes which drain urine produced by the kidneys down to the bladder; the bladder itself; and the urethra, the tube which drains it to the outside. Inadequate drainage or blockage of the system in foetal or early life can dramatically interfere with kidney development. Urological surgery is aimed at correcting such problems. The associated limitation of kidney function and predisposition to infection requires careful management, which I now took on.

While the numbers of renal patients grew, a considerable proportion of my time was taken up by general medical paediatrics. I was responsible for all admissions and emergencies on one night each week and one weekend each month. I was also available for renal consultation 24-7. The lessons learnt across these two areas of responsibility were complementary.

Gradually, I became aware of how families measure up a doctor. They are alert to how a consultant behaves towards both children and adults. Parents look for competence and compassion in those who treat their children. Recognising specialist expertise and knowledge gives them confidence and helps allay their fears. The children respond best to kindness, gentleness and a little bit of fun. Adopting these skills and attitudes, even subconsciously, determines the level of trust that develops.

Talitha

The neonatal and post cardiac surgery intensive care units soon began to call for advice and assistance with the management of patients with impaired kidney function. Early treatment of acute kidney injury improved outcomes and quickly became embedded as a routine part of my work.

Pushing open the door to the Cardiac unit, it was noticeable that the majority of the patients were adults recovering from conditions such as coronary artery bypass, or heart valve replacement surgery. Isolated in one corner on the right lay two or three patients at the other end of the age spectrum. Operating to correct congenital structural cardiac problems is a very special skill. This surgery may be performed on a heart not much bigger than a large adult thumb, while the baby's circulation is maintained by a heart bypass pump, which temporarily takes over that particular function of the heart. When the circulation is precarious, the blood supply to the kidneys may be reduced by the body's innate protective systems in order to maintain the blood supply to critical organs, such as the brain and lungs. The kidneys may take some time to recover after the normal circulation is restored. On occasions the cardiac surgeon would call on me to initiate a short period of dialysis to reduce the fluid overload on the heart caused by little or no urine output.At other times the treatment might also be required to correct abnormal blood biochemistry, such as a high level of potassium, caused by its inadequate removal by the kidneys. This can cause irregularities in heart rhythm or even precipitate a cardiac arrest. Before intervening we both needed to sit down with the already highly stressed and anxious parents to explain what we proposed. This task is as important as the dialysis process itself. I was a new face to the parents, but they often had a special relationship with the surgeon, the medical cardiologists or the neonatologists. I explained the reasons for the intervention and what it entailed, not over-playing the risks, but admitting that success was not always assured. When we delivered the information together as a team, it meant the parents' faith did not rest solely with one individual.

On one occasion, reviewing a baby who had come through such a crisis, I asked a question I had suppressed while she was very ill.

"Your little girl has quite an unusual name. Even working in London and Manchester I have never met anyone called Talitha. Do you mind me asking where it comes from?"

They reminded me of a story in the Bible about a rich man called Jarius, who approached Jesus and begged him to come and see his daughter, who was extremely sick. As Jesus arrived at his house, people came out to say it was too late. The child was already dead, they said. Jesus told them she was not dead but sleeping, he entered the house, took her hand and said, "Little girl arise". In Aramaic, they explained, this phrase translates as, "Talitha Cumi."

They looked at each other and the infant.

"Our little girl was close to death when she was born, but she survived in answer to our prayers, so we chose that name."

An imaginary friend

I was sometimes reminded that I was still learning the art of doctoring and discovered unforeseen responsibilities. Parents sometimes believe doctors have special powers beyond their medical expertise. Powers of which I was unaware.

One afternoon, I was in my outpatient clinic dictating a letter for a family doctor about the patient I had just seen. I added a few supplementary thoughts into the clinical notes, while wondering if there was any chance I might have a few free minutes to grab a coffee, now that it was almost 4 p.m.. There was a tentative knock at the door and a pause. The nurses usually knocked, but then just came on in, so I finished writing. The knock came again, a little harder this time. I walked over and opened the door. The mother of a six-year-old boy, edged past me. I knew her well as a warm, friendly woman, with a ready smile. She and her boy had the same sunny temperament. Today she seemed less relaxed than usual.

"I wondered if I could have a quick word with you before Johnny comes in?" she asked apologetically.

"Of course," I replied, shaking her hand. I asked if there was some new worry, or whether he had become more unwell since their last visit. I led her to a seat beside my desk. I never sat behind it, so I pulled my chair closer to hers and tried to guess from her face how big the problem might be.

"Oh, John's fine. It's nothing to do with his treatment or anything like that. I wondered if you could help us with some worrying behaviour which we have been trying to sort out. His dad and I feel we are getting nowhere at the minute - and because our boy thinks of you as a very important person, we thought a word from you might get through to him. He actually likes coming to see you at the hospital, you know?" Then she added, with a little laugh, "Of course it does mean he gets a half day off school!"

I was intrigued. She hesitated and began to explain that I probably knew where she lived, not far from the hospital. I nodded. She added that I might not realise that the main north-to-south railway line ran directly behind their back garden.

Recently neighbours had told her some boys had been seen running chicken across the tracks. Apparently some older lads had bent some of the bars of a substantial metal fence protecting the railway. The opening in the fence near their home created a dangerous shortcut to the football stadium and pitches beyond. She took a deep breath. "Our Johnny has always been fascinated by the trains and knows not to go too close. Ever since he was a toddler, he has loved to stand in the garden and watch the Dublin express rush past. The noise never seemed to bother him. Recently, one of our neighbours caught Johnny trying to get through the fence and stopped him. It has scared me to death. So his dad and I sat him down and had a serious talk. We asked Johnny if he had ever gone near the track. He denied that he ever has done so. When we pressed him and said someone was sure they had seen him there, he told us he would never go through the fence, but George was a bad boy, and he had done it. This really frightened us because George is his invisible friend!"

I could see that his mum had gone a little pale as she talked and was struggling to get a tissue from her handbag.

"Johnny has an imaginary friend who is getting the blame?" I asked.

"Yes, he doesn't talk about him a lot - but when he is playing on his own with his cars or toys, I sometimes hear him talking to George. At bedtime he occasionally mentions doing things with George that day. He doesn't really claim George is a real boy. In fact, I am fairly sure he knows he is just make believe. We have brought up the danger of the train track several times but each time he says George is the bad boy who goes there."

She gave me an anxious look.

"Do you think you could say something to Johnny? I think he would listen to you".

My first thought was that I hoped someone had alerted the Railway Company so they could repair the fence - but I agreed to help with a furrowed brow, not sure of what I might say, but promised to give it some thought. I realised this was possibly a more difficult problem than most of the medical ones I had dealt with so far that afternoon.

After I dealt with another patient, the Ritchie family came in. I had a half-formed plan. Johnny bounced into my room, happy and bright as usual, ready for a chat and a bit of good-natured banter. He had a mischievous sense of humour. I discussed his medical situation with his mum then, as I examined him and checked his blood pressure, our talk turned to football. He was like his dad, an avid Liverpool supporter. I pretended to be a United fan, to his disgust. I casually asked if he had ever been to a match at the big stadium near his house. He told me that his dad had promised to take him to a match for his birthday. I pointed out he would have to go over the footbridge above the railway to get there and he agreed. I mentioned it was the only safe way get across because of the trains. We talked about how exciting it was to stand on the footbridge as the trains rush past underneath. His eyes lit up as we talked. Then, changing to a more serious tone, I told him a story.

"A while ago we had an injured boy brought to the hospital who had thought he might try to get a closer look at the engine as it sped past." I explained that what many people did not know was that if you were to stand too close to a fast train, the blast of wind as it rushes past can knock a boy over and even suck them in towards the wheels.

"Luckily," I said, "that boy, called George, wasn't badly hurt and just needed some cuts stitched and bandaged up and, I think, a strong plaster for his arm. He has never ever gone near a railway line again, unless he is going on a train trip - and then he makes sure to hold on tightly to his mum or dad's hand." I smiled and tickled Johnny under the chin. "Remember that and be very careful if you ever travel by train to see Liverpool play!"

I turned to his mum, "It's lucky you have such a clever boy, even if he supports that team. I bet he knows how dangerous trains can be. I'm glad to say he looks the picture of health today, so I do not need to see him again for several months."

When I did see him again the message seemed to have got through and there was no mention of George or the railway on that visit.

A poke in the eye

Christmas Day at home. The crescendo of excitement on Christmas Eve meant that both Anne and I, and indeed our children, had despaired that anyone would ever get to sleep. Then suddenly, it seemed it was morning. We pulled back the curtains a little in an effort to persuade the kids it was still very early and dark outside - but they had discovered the stockings hung on the end of their beds were full and so were already bouncing down the stairs, trailing them behind. They were certain Santa had been.

"Yes! Yes!" they whooped, "The lemonade, biscuits and carrots we left out before going to bed are gone!"

It was true. Only a few strategic crumbs remained.

They began tearing the bright wrapping paper from the presents that had magically appeared overnight.

By early afternoon, as we waited for the traditional roast turkey dinner to be ready, we watched Top Of The Pops on TV, showing the hit songs of the past year. I snatched up my toddler daughter and danced with her in my arms to a favourite number. Spirits were high and we all laughed as we tried to sing along. She shrieked with delight and waved her arms in the air in time to the beat, as my son skipped around us. Their mum swayed to the music, her thoughts half on how things were progressing in the kitchen.

A sharp pain shot through my right eye and I blinked tears away. When the music faded, I felt the full effect of the tiny fingernail which had accidentally scored across the pupil. As the next Christmas rock song started up, I struggled a tissue out of my pocket, dabbing at the tears now streaming down my face. After a few more numbers there was no improvement and I set my daughter down.

"Anne, will you take a look at my eye? Can you see anything in it? I got a finger in the eye, horsing around just now, but it feels as if a piece of grit or something has been left behind."

"My goodness," she said, perhaps using a slightly stronger expletive. "Your entire eyeball is red and inflamed. What on earth have you done?"

I explained what had happened. She told me to follow her into the kitchen so that, unhindered by children, she could get a better look. I followed obediently. After finding no foreign body there, she removed an

200

egg cup from a cupboard. She lifted the kettle, in which she had recently boiled water. The cup was washed, then rinsed out and filled with sterile water. A towel was draped over my shoulder.

"Press the egg cup around your eye and hold it tightly against your eyelids."

I did as instructed by the family nurse.

"Now tilt your head right back, open your eye wide and let the warm water bathe it. Blink your eye lid open, then shut, several times. That should wash out any grit and calm down the irritation."

The children appeared to watch, wanting to know what was going on. We explained dad's eye was sore and mum was helping to make it better.

The eye continued to be uncomfortable and watering, although bathing it several times helped. Eventually, as dinner was served and everyone sat down, shiny Christmas crackers were pulled with satisfying explosions. Out fell party hats and tiny trinkets, puzzles, key rings and in my case, incredibly, a black pirate's eyepatch. This provoked great hilarity, mixed with some sympathy. I joined in the merriment around the table. My eye still had not settled and I slipped away for a few moments, found some gauze in our medicine chest, pressed it against my closed eye and held it firmly in place with the eyepatch. I knew this would prevent me from blinking and protect my cornea from any further abrasive eyelid movement. I returned to the table, pretending to the children that this was all part of the fun of the day. If my eye remained sore and inflamed by the morning, I planned to have it examined at the hospital.

The paediatric intensive care unit was busy that Boxing Day, with all but one of the ventilator spaces occupied when I arrived. Once the essential decisions were made, the work of the morning completed and the ward round finished, a colleague had a look at my eye and prescribed antibiotic ointment. I called in at our accident and emergency department and they provided me with a more professional replacement for my pirate eyepatch. As the day progressed, my eye began to feel better but late in the evening an unconscious, critically ill infant was admitted with a high temperature. The baby was having multiple seizures and we suspected a diagnosis of meningitis or encephalitis. It was imperative that I started intravenous treatment and performed a lumbar puncture. Anticonvulsant drugs controlled the fits and we elected to put the infant on full life support to prevent any damage from possible brain swelling. I explained to the young parents the reasons for everything we were doing. They sat holding rosary beads, praying, a finger in the baby's hand.

A few hours later, the initial drip line in the back of the hand began to leak into the surrounding tissues. I had difficulty inserting a new cannula into a tiny vein to continue the treatment, acutely aware of the parents silently watching. Normally, I had little problem with such a procedure, but after the frustration of two failed attempts, I admitted to myself that my difficulty was with focusing on the task with one eye. I stepped aside and pulled off the bandage and tried again. This was not much help, as a renewed flood of tears distorted my sight.

Making a rapid decision, I opened the drug cupboard, located some lignocaine anaesthetic eye drops, retired to the office and dropped two or three of these into my damaged eye. The discomfort, irritation and tear production gradually eased away. I returned to the baby and within minutes the cannula was in place and the drug infusion was running again. Relieved, I reapplied the bandage.

By morning the baby was stable. I tentatively removed the bandage to check my eye in the mirror. I discovered the eyelid looked swollen and, when opened, my eye looked really angry. I phoned the on-call ophthalmologist and she agreed to see me immediately. She introduced some fluorescein drops into my eye in order to stain and reveal any surface damage. She also applied some atropine, a drug that would block the pupillary muscle spasm that was causing the pain. My eye was carefully examined using a slit lamp instrument, which produces a narrow vertical light beam. She moved the beam slowly across the surface of my pupil while focusing on my cornea. She sighed gently, sat back and shook her head.

"I'm afraid you have an extensive corneal abrasion. It's the worst I've ever seen from a simple scratch from a child's finger."

At this point I confessed to using the lignocaine, as I sat with my chin on the support shelf of the slit lamp device. This made it difficult to avoid looking directly at her.

She looked back with disbelief.

"You should have known that was not very clever," she scolded. "I was going to say your daughter must have very long nails which need to be trimmed at once if you or her mum haven't done so already. In fact, it seems it's her dad who needs to be more careful and avoid treating himself and endangering his sight.

"I'm afraid that as a result of what you have done, with the best of intentions, I'm sure, you are going to need your eye bandaged for a week at least, except when administering the drops I am going to prescribe. I will need to see you again in 48 hours. I expect your cornea will heal gradually, but you may be left prone to recurrent corneal erosions."

I was beginning to feel like a fool.

"With your eye anaesthetised, you couldn't feel the damage you were doing when no protective tears were produced. With a dry eye and no sensation, you were probably stripping off a little more corneal surface epithelium each time you blinked until the feeling returned."

I found myself apologising profusely. Walking away, I admitted to myself that the pragmatic decision, taken in the emotion of the moment, had ignored the potential risk. Still, my patient was stable and her brain was protected, giving the antimicrobials a chance to take effect.

As it turned out my cornea healed quickly - but that eye remained hypersensitive forever. Even the smallest amount of sunscreen lotion getting into it leaves me streaming tears for hours. One compensation was that, by the time my eye recovered, so had the tiny patient.

After my daughter managed to stab her finger in my eye again about six months later, Anne became convinced that I had a defective blink reflex, reinforcing my colleague's view that the whole episode was completely my own fault.

A breakdown in communication

Despite considerable demands on my time, I was approached to temporarily fill a gap at the child development clinic. The consultant there was leaving to work abroad. I had limited experience in early childhood developmental problems but, on meeting the other members of the team, I was reassured by their expertise and agreed to join them for a weekly assessment clinic until a new specialist could be appointed.

In the course of a morning, each child had a full clinical examination, generally concentrating on the neurological system. There was also an assessment by a specialist developmental physiotherapist; an occupational therapist; and some time with a child psychologist and our social worker, who both offered family support. The first thing I learnt from Dama, the senior physiotherapist, was how important it was to treat our little patients like any baby, whatever their level of disability. I noticed how she sat each one on her knee as we listened to their parents' concerns. I soon was following her example, conveying a message in this non-verbal way that we knew how precious their baby was, and that we wanted to help in every way we could.

I also learnt that most of the morning would be spent sitting on the floor watching how the children played.

Mothers sometimes told us that, once it became known their baby had a problem such as Down's Syndrome, some people avoided them, even crossing the street to do so. This was undoubtedly hurtful - sometimes driven by a fear of saying the wrong thing, perhaps, but ultimately having the same effect. Patricia, the psychologist in the team, listened carefully and ventured helpful advice.

Early on, I was reminded of how difficult it was to communicate bad news sensitively.

After a careful assessment of a little boy, it fell to me to tell the parents that we believed the reason he could not yet stand or walk was related to problems during his birth. We believed that a period of hypoxia had resulted in a brain injury and a degree of cerebral palsy, a condition affecting his muscle function and coordination. Dama followed up with a demonstration of a series of daily exercises which she believed would improve his muscle function so that he would eventually walk.

A month later we reviewed the boy's progress. As we did so, I talked gently about the problems faced by children with cerebral palsy. His mother broke down, shocked and tearful.

"Cerebral palsy?" she sobbed. "Why did no one mention this at our last visit when his dad was with me?"

We spent a long time consoling her and trying to emphasise the positive things we identified in her little boy. Dama had an innate kindness and an ability to transfer some of her optimism to the most anxious of mothers. Later, our social worker sat talking with the mother over a cup of coffee, as her baby played on the exercise mat with another physiotherapist. We offered to contact her husband, who was at work. Eventually she was able to compose herself and left with a promise from the social worker that she would visit her at home before the end of the week.

Later, feeling I had let down the mother and the team, I asked, "How did that happen? I remember mentioning cerebral palsy last time. The diagnosis is in my notes and in the letter we sent to the family doctor." Chastened and humbled, I appealed for confirmation and support.

Dama, with long experience, reassured me that she had seen this happen before. She reminded me that on occasions when some dreaded or shocking diagnosis is delivered or confirmed, only the initial words of the discussion are remembered. She talked about how people's minds might go blank so that very little is taken in - and how this response could be triggered even before a professional began speaking, by taking in their demeanour alone.

I acknowledged that this was true. I had seen this same reaction in the adult wards, when the word cancer was mentioned. I now appreciated it might occur in many situations. I became be alert to the reality that when, in my daily work, I used phrases like, kidney damage, kidney failure, dialysis, or kidney transplant, these were equally scary terms, that needed careful explanation and time to be assimilated.

I wondered how we might circumvent such communication failure at the developmental clinic. After discussion, we concluded we needed to start each conversation with positive messages and gradually build up to any conclusion which might be upsetting. For disappointing diagnoses, it would be best to speak to both parents together or, if there was only one, to suggest they were accompanied by a supportive friend or relative. We needed to arrange early follow-up appointments, and pre-plan contact with supportive community networks and charities.

One practical innovation we initiated was to obtain a video camera so that we could give parents a recording on tape to take home, showing the exercises we recommended, based on our clinical analysis, and including some supportive positive advice.

Distraught or dangerous

The phone rang on my secretary's desk. Mary looked at me over the top of her electronic typewriter and at the pile of letters which I had been signing, from my general medical clinic. She had expertly produced them, having discreetly corrected the grammatical and other errors in my dictation. She was eager to get them to the post. She picked up the handset and listened before handing it to me. The relatives of a child who had died overnight, after a prolonged illness, had arrived at the ward to collect a Death Certificate. As I headed there, I prepared myself to be compassionate, understanding and kind, knowing how emotional our meeting would be. The father introduced me to the family members who had come along to offer him their support. We sat for some time and talked about their little girl and not just of her illness. I heard about her first steps, first words, her love of singing, her playfulness when well, and how she was always ready to give and receive a cuddle. Eventually I produced the Certificate and explained the terminology. These were tearful moments. Finally we shook hands again, and they left, their lives changed forever.

I sat alone in the small ward office feeling drained and saddened. I inevitably thought of more difficult situations I had faced after a child had been lost. Again I felt the anguished grief of a single mother who refused to be parted from her baby for hours, but sat swaying back and forth, as she nursed her tiny infant, resistant to reasoning. Eventually the situation was resolved by a gracious clergyman who sat with her for some time before encouraging her to join with him in a goodbye prayer.

I went over in my mind a day, when I was urgently called to a ward because a bereaved father had arrived, desperately upset. I was told that he was beside himself with his loss, throwing furniture across the floor and punching the wall. When I arrived in the unit, the ward Sister was waiting, and led me quickly to a side ward. As we approached, one of the hospital security staff intercepted me.

"You'd better not go in, Doc," he said. "I tried to talk to him, but he virtually threw me out of the room. He has half wrecked the place. The nurses are terrified, so I've locked the door until he calms down, poor guy."

I tentatively looked through the glass panel in the door, and my white coat was spotted. The father was shouting something incoherently, which I could not hear. He was a big, heavy man, almost six foot tall, and still in his outdoor work clothes. I explained that it was imperative that I spoke with him.

The security officer looked at me and understood. He nodded his head sadly. "I'll be out here if you need me."

Carefully, he opened the door and I stepped inside.

The father rushed towards me and I involuntarily braced myself. He threw big strong arms around me and fell onto my shoulders. He was shaking, sobbing and weeping. I wrapped my arms around him and, with difficulty, held him up. He was saying,

"What went wrong? What will we do without him?"

I managed to help him onto a chair and righted another which had been knocked over. I sat down beside him while he gathered himself. He slumped over with his head in his hands. I wiped my own eyes, and tried to explain what had happened, and how we had tried to save his boy. I could feel the pain he was suffering, but there was nothing more I could do for now, except sit with him.

The door opened quietly. It was the ward orderly. She held a tray with a pot of tea, two cups and a plate of plain Marie biscuits. I was so grateful for her typical thoughtfulness and kindness. I began to talk softly, offering sympathy, trying to explain again what might have caused the tragedy.

None of us would forget those tragic days..

Important groundwork

I arranged a series of meetings with the surgeons who performed kidney transplants in adult patients. There were, of course, no paediatric surgeons with transplantation experience in Belfast, nor indeed in many major centres.

After several weeks of discussion we agreed that, initially, only school-age children weighing 20 kilograms or more should be accepted to the transplant programme. We would reconsider this limitation when we had all gained more experience. I suggested involving some of the paediatric surgeons with operative urological experience to assist at the transplants, thus utilising two areas of expertise. The idea was welcomed, so I approached my paediatric surgical colleagues and, after gaining their agreement, we had a tentative plan in place. The hospital anaesthetists on the adult transplant team confirmed they had experience with anaesthetising children and were happy to be involved. I gained the ready agreement of the adult transplant unit to accept the children postoperatively, with the understanding that I would always be available for both management and advice.

I reviewed in detail the published immune suppressive protocols for kidney transplants in children. Then, in discussion with the adult nephrologists, I drew up a variation on what was called "The Belfast Recipe". Dr Mollie McGeown, who set up the adult unit, had championed an approach that employed lower doses of steroid and other immunosuppressive drugs compared to previous regimens, and had demonstrated its efficacy in preventing rejection of the new organs. We believed this would be equally effective, yet produce fewer side effects, in children. The lower dose of steroids involved was an attractive proposition. They were a key component of the cocktail of anti-rejection drugs that prevent a donated organ from failing, but had the potential to inhibit normal growth in proportion to the dosage given. We had now an agreed approach and guidelines to follow.

The adult service had begun to offer Chronic Ambulatory Peritoneal Dialysis (CAPD) to some adults as an alternative to hospital-based machine haemodialysis. I have mentioned that I had been attracted to this form of therapy when in Manchester. It had the advantage that children could be treated at home and continue with normal schooling and lead more normal lives. I now had the opportunity to work with the local CAPD nursing team to develop this option for children. I worried that they might find this a daunting prospect, having no experience of child patients, but once they met my young friends and their families, they rose magnificently to the challenge. Joyce, Brid, Joanne, Susan, Joan, and others all took the children to their hearts and, almost as importantly, won the trust of their parents.

We were now all ready to embark on a new journey together - families, nurses, anaesthetists, surgeons and myself - knowing that it should lead to a new or prolonged life for children with renal failure.

Home dialysis treatment

Most families were understandably apprehensive when we first suggested the possibility of home dialysis. They would, after all, become responsible for the day-to-day treatment of their child. The idea that the lining of the abdomen, the peritoneum, could filter waste material from the blood circulating inside the child's body must have seemed unbelievable at first. First, each family home was assessed to determine if some plumbing or other minor alterations were required to facilitate the dialysis and to identify adequate space to store the sterile fluid packs. We tried to prepare parents well in advance, and none ever refused to take on the task. We also spent considerable time preparing the children. Meeting an adult patient who already performed their own dialysis was helpful and we had no problem finding volunteers. This preparation became easier once there were several children on the programme who could meet and reassure those who were about to start. I was heartened by the mutual support I saw between families. One mother, normally a shy person, readily agreed to take part in a video demonstrating the dialysis procedure and the importance of the aseptic "non touch" technique designed to prevent infection.

A few weeks before a patient was due to start dialysis, the surgeon placed a soft catheter through a small incision in the anaesthetised child's tummy, sliding it deep into the abdominal cavity. The first thing the parents learnt was how to care for the skin around the exit site, which has to be cleaned each day. The wound was then allowed to heal for a couple of weeks so that a tight seal formed around the catheter and its teflon cuff, which became embedded in the abdominal wall. Over the next few weeks the parents worked with the nurses, learning how to safely connect the bags of dialysis fluid to this tube. Using this technique, the fluid was run in and left for several hours before being drained back out into the empty bag. Cleanliness is of paramount importance in order to avoid the possibility of inflammation caused by germs entering the system. Hand washing is essential before the catheter is touched at each step. This requires good bathroom facilities, so we arranged financial support to fund bathroom alterations if these proved necessary, often from charitable funds.

During the training period at hospital, the volume and type of fluid which would achieve the best results for an individual child was determined. The daily weight and the amount of fluid the child drank and passed out each day was factored into this calculation.

Both parents usually undertook the training or, if that was difficult, another family member or close friend would come along to help. This ensured a backup was available if one person became unwell or needed a break.

When the parents became confident enough, they performed the dialysis alone in the hospital overnight with no nurses involved, although nearby to provide help if needed.

Then it was time to move home. One of the nurses stayed at the house on the first evening but took no part in the treatment unless they were called upon. Next, it was into a routine of three or more bag changes each day. If the blood biochemistry and fluid balance permitted, a day off each week was sanctioned.

The stolen bicycle

As the number of children being treated increased, a weekly paediatric clinic was established at the adult dialysis day unit. I regularly cycled the mile or two between the Children's Hospital and City Hospital campus where it was sited, and where the initial training took place. On each visit, I padlocked my bicycle to a drainpipe just outside the entrance door. One day I left the one-storey building to find that the plastic drainpipe was smashed and the bicycle gone. It was a relatively small irritation, offset by the success of the fledgling programme.

The mother of one of the first children to start on the CAPD programme was by chance, a qualified nurse. She, of course, understood and practised aseptic techniques in the course of her own work, so she coped easily with our rules for avoiding infection when carrying out the dialysis. She was well acquainted with connecting and disconnecting intravenous lines, not a dissimilar procedure to attaching PD fluid lines to the peritoneal catheter. The expertise she already possessed made her training relatively straightforward and enabled the team to gain confidence before taking on further patients. This family travelled quite a distance to the clinic, so her husband chose to drive and attend each appointment.

One day, I noticed he was not present. After reviewing her son, David, and his home dialysis record, we chatted while waiting for the local anaesthetic cream to numb the skin on his arm, before taking the routine blood test. I remarked to his mother on the father's absence. She informed me that he was actually waiting outside in the car and asked if I would mind slipping out to talk to him.

"Could he not come in as usual?" I asked, a little puzzled.

"He has something he wants to talk to you about, privately, away from everyone," she explained, clearly anxious that I sought him out.

"You can't miss him. He'll be in the blue estate car just at the door. He'll be watching out for you."

Mystified, but having great respect for her, I agreed.

As I exited the building, I saw him climb out of the car and walk around to its rear. As I reached him, he swung up the hatchback door, and battled to extract a red road bike.

"We heard you had your bike stolen and our boy suggested we got you a replacement."

I was stunned and became slightly incoherent as I thanked him for this amazing generosity. I looked around and found his son, his wife, and a couple of the nurses had appeared, all smiling and laughing, clearly in on the surprise. I hugged each in turn. This was a special gift coming from people in the midst of what was undoubtedly the most worrying time of their lives. The much-prized bicycle was to be used for many years to come. I made sure it was never stolen.

The call

One morning in 1982, my radio pager went off, the bleep pattern alerting me to an urgent message.

I contacted the hospital switchboard.

"We are holding a call from the UK transplant service in Bristol. Can you take it?"

For each new renal failure patient, there are detailed discussions with the chief scientist in the laboratory regarding the tissue-type profile they have identified from the blood samples we have provided. With the scientist's advice, a decision is made as to the level of tissue match or mismatch we would accept for the individual. Certain tissue type mismatches are known to be more likely to trigger a rejection reaction in a particular patient. A single mismatch against a common tissue type in the population may initially be acceptable if it is judged unlikely to stimulate a strong immune reaction. However, this choice can render the patient permanently sensitised to that tissue type. This would exclude any kidney with that tissue type from use in a second transplant, should that be necessary in years to come. This information was explained to the parents and to the child, depending on their age. Having confirmed that they understood the risks and benefits of a transplant, and were keen to proceed, we placed their child on call for a donor organ, registering the patient's name and details with the UK Transplant Service. The tissue type of every donated organ is also registered with UKTS when offered. The national computer can identify from the central list, the individual with the closest tissue match to the donated kidney. When a child's kidney was donated, it was preferentially offered to the closest matching child on the list, before even being offered to an adult.

The call was put through to me.

"Good morning doctor, we wish to offer you a kidney which we believe to be an excellent match for one of your patients."

I carefully noted down the information about the donor and kidney, specifically the tissue type breakdown, but including the cause and time of the donor's death, their size, age, medical history, the anatomy of the kidney and its vessels, and location of the hospital from which it was to be transported.

I carefully compared the two tissue types, and felt a mixture of pleasure, excitement and apprehension.

"Thank you, I would like to provisionally accept the kidney and will confirm within the hour or sooner

212

I hung up and discarded my plans for the morning. First, I phoned the parents to inform them a suitable kidney may have become available and checked they were still happy to go ahead with the surgery. The next call was to the transplant surgeon. He was already in the operating theatre block but able to come to the phone between cases. I shared all the details with him and confirmed he would be free to operate later if needed. He agreed the organ, tissue type and recipient size were suitable. He took on the responsibility of arranging an operating theatre and alerting the anaesthetist. When I spoke to the renal unit they confirmed there was an available bed. I contacted a paediatric surgeon who agreed to assist with the transplant and, finally, called back to the UKTS, confirming our acceptance of the kidney.

"The kidney will be on the next flight to Belfast International Airport," they told me. "We estimate it should arrive with you around 1.30 p.m.. All the transfer arrangements are in place."

I next called our own tissue typing laboratory to arrange a tissue cross match. This is a similar, but more complex, process to matching blood for a transfusion. It would take around six hours. We now had a provisional start time for surgery. I called back the parents, who had taken their son out of school, and asked them to bring him to the unit at one o'clock to have blood samples taken. I explained there would then be up to a six-hour wait for the cross match results to come through, during which time he would not be able to eat, prior to the anaesthetic being administered. There was just time for him to have some light food, perhaps something that he really liked, before they left home.

"This is the day we have been waiting for," came the reply. "Our bag is packed. We have his favourite lunch ready, but I doubt if we will be able to eat anything ourselves."

"Best to try, it may be a long and tiring day ahead."

I let the dialysis nurses know what was happening before I headed for my regular outpatient clinic. They already knew. The hospital grapevine was in full working order. We were all a little tense. It was an important and anxious day for the family and the apprehension was shared by us all. The parents and nurses endeavoured to amuse and distract the little boy while we all waited.

After the last outpatient left, I was dictating some letters when my pager bleeped again. It was the scientist in the tissue-typing laboratory.

"It's good news," she said. "There is no reaction by the patient's cells against the donor tissue. We have used today's blood samples and stored historic ones from previous clinic visits. No reaction shows up on any of the tests. I guess it's all systems go. I am really pleased for him, I will think of nothing else tonight. I hope all goes well."

I informed the surgeon and the rest of the team and went to the family to explain the sequence of events from there. They had talked with the surgeon and anaesthetist and were hiding their anxiety to stop it being transmitted to their boy, who was also putting on a brave face. He told me that his last trip to the operating theatre hadn't been as bad as he had feared. I reflected inwardly that this surgery would be a bigger job than fitting a dialysis catheter as I smiled encouragement. It was as if he was trying to protect his mum and dad by acting like he was okay with everything. He was an eight-year-old anyone could have been proud of. I was, as ever, impressed by the courage of my young friends.

As the physician, I was not involved in the surgery but could not resist changing into scrubs later, and discreetly calling into the operating theatre. I was able to report back to the parents that all was going to plan.

Morning came. There had been no problems during three hours in the operating theatre, or overnight since. The bladder drainage bag by the bedside contained an impressive volume of urine. The monitors showed a normal temperature, regular heartbeat and stable blood pressure. The biochemistry results, which had just come back from the laboratory, showed a significant improvement on those taken before the surgery.

The new kidney was working.

The patient was asleep, thanks to the analgesia prescribed by the anaesthetist to counteract any pain. His parents were exhausted, but the success so far had buoyed them up and raised the morale of the whole ward.

I was enormously pleased and relieved but knew we would need to be vigilant in the days and weeks ahead. The immunosuppressive drugs which counteract any tendency for the new kidney to be rejected also reduce resistance to infection - so meticulous attention to fluid balance, wound management and pain relief were among several of many newly-crucial tasks.

I thought of the donor family as I left the ward, hoping that, by now, their sorrow would be tempered a little by their gift of life to another child. I felt relieved and thankful that all had gone well so far and that, at last, the renal replacement programme for children was fully up and running. I had spent two years since I was appointed developing a structure and building a fledgling team to deliver the service. It was almost 12 years since a little girl had inspired me to become a paediatrician, and more than five years since another little girl with progressive kidney disease fired my determination to become a renal specialist.

A message from the H blocks

One morning, as I moved from room to room reviewing each patient's progress, I found one little girl who had recently received a new kidney, still fast asleep. A nurse whispered, "She has been very restless and was crying for her dad in the middle of the night. He was unable to come to the hospital, so she only settled a couple of hours ago when one of the night staff she likes, sat with her for an hour."

The girl's observations and urine output were fine, so I decided to leave examining her until later. I noticed she had many get well soon cards at her bedside. I picked a couple up. One was from her primary school class, signed in wobbly handwriting by every pupil. The next one was also crowded with signatures under the heading: "From your Uncle Barny and all the lads in the H Block."

The segregated H blocks in the Maze prison held men suspected or convicted of involvement in the troubles and civil unrest. It was easy to forget that these people, some interned without a trial, had families like everyone else, some of whom might be seriously ill. They were not exempt from ordinary worries.

When I dropped into her side ward again later in the week, she was happily playing a board game with her dad. As I left, he called me aside.

"Doc, I couldn't get up to see my wee girl that night when she was so upset. I didn't want to run the gauntlet of police checkpoints. You see, I haven't been able to afford the tax and insurance for my old car but in the morning, when I heard how upset she had been, I took a chance and drove here. It was just my luck to be pulled over half a mile from the hospital. I've been reported for driving without tax and I have to produce my insurance certificate at Andytown police station. Thank God, the police let me drive on into the hospital when I explained my little girl was critically ill. There's a chance they might drop the charge if you would write something supportive on my behalf."

He looked at me hopefully.

Shortly, I sat down to dictate a letter. I never enquired whether he subsequently taxed and insured the car.

Ten out of ten

Because the early transplants took place in the adult unit, my days started and finished there. Typically, I arrived at 7.30 a.m. to check on any child whose operation had taken place in the previous few days. I took the high-speed staff lift to the eleventh floor of possibly the ugliest building in Belfast. The changing room was usually silent and empty as I undressed and put on a blue surgical vest and trousers, taken from a freshly laundered pile. I added a protective theatre hat and overshoes and stepped over the red line on the floor, which marked the demarcation line between the rest of the hospital and the clean environment of the transplant suite.

On one such morning, a staff nurse joined me in a young patient's room, "He has been a perfect boy, and his morning blood tests are already dispatched to the laboratory. His urine output is picking up and, as you know, last night's results showed an early improvement."

I smiled a greeting to his mum. The patient remained half awake as I washed my hands. I talked to them both quietly as I examined him.

"Do I have to have a needle for blood tests?" he asked.

"No, love, a sample has already been taken from the cannula in your arm while you were asleep," his nurse explained with a smile. He looked at his arm and, pleased, smiled weakly back. I bantered with him gently about his favourite football team and told him he was the bravest boy in the

216

hospital. Someone appeared at the door of his room with a printout of the laboratory results.

"These are looking really good, even better than last night. His new kidney is kicking in, although it is early days."

"This calls for a glass of champagne," said his dad.

"No," his mum disagreed with a grin. "Let's settle for a few glasses of wee."

There had now been 10 successive and successful paediatric transplants since we set off on this quest.

15. Moving ahead

Within a few years, a hospital and home peritoneal dialysis and successful kidney transplantation programme for school age children became established. There had been invaluable support from the adult unit, where the early transplant operations were performed. Nevertheless, I was acutely aware that ideally young patients should be cared for in a paediatric environment. The time came when we were sufficiently experienced and ready to move. The Children's Hospital had a particular expertise. Its qualified children's nurses were specifically trained to manage ill babies, toddlers and young children of all ages. They had experience of coping with stressed-out parents and distressed children. Paediatric dieticians, social workers and child psychologists were part of the team. In the outpatient clinics and the radiology department, friendly staff were tolerant of those who are apprehensive or upset. For inpatients there was a hospital school providing bedside or classroom education. Play therapists helped younger ones cope with hospital stays and treatment. Visiting hours for parents and grandparents were unrestricted.

The paediatric consultants specialised in every aspect of childhood disease. These included, for example, an endocrinologist, who could advise on optimising children's growth when it was restricted by renal impairment. There was an infectious disease specialist - a valuable asset as transplanted children were especially vulnerable to bacterial and childhood infections including chicken pox and measles. This susceptibility was due to the immunosuppressive, anti-rejection drugs, and should any infection develop it needed expert aggressive management. Crucially, the hospital had a paediatric intensive care unit for immediate post-transplant care.

The adult renal unit had a different expertise. It had the best renal replacement programme and results in the UK. Sharing that skill and expertise was vital in building the same standard of treatment for children with renal failure. Parents appreciated the special efforts staff made to accommodate the needs of children who had surgery there and who received their post-transplant care in the unit's isolation rooms. On a personal level, I found the team invariably supportive and professional in working with me

218

as the visiting paediatric nephrologist. The treatment of children with every kidney disease was performed in the children's hospital. Unfortunately for a few, terminal renal failure developed and transplantation surgery was then scheduled for the adult unit. At that point I continued to coordinate their care while leaning on the experience and facilities of the adult team. This approach had been rewarded with early success. The longer-term aim was to gradually transfer all that treatment, including the necessary surgery, to the children's hospital. This was now feasible, as our confidence and experience had grown. I had no shame in poaching one of the best dialysis nurses to help achieve the transition. The implementation of the plan was accelerated when three babies, in rapid succession, were born with a congenital nephrotic syndrome. This is a rare genetic condition occurring in only one in 100,000 births. There is no curative treatment, as the kidney filtering structure fails to develop in the normal way before birth. In those days, children with this condition often died in infancy and those who survived developed renal failure around the age of two.

I formulated an aggressive treatment plan. The hope was that with dialysis and a new kidney, they would survive beyond their third birthday, leading to a reasonably normal childhood. After consulting colleagues in other paediatric centres, I concluded that, technically, transplantation was most likely to be successful once children reached about 10 kilograms in weight - about the average weight for an 18-month-old toddler. Infants with congenital nephrotic syndrome have massive urinary protein loss, which, in many, exceeds their calorie and protein intake. Important proteins which the body produces to fight infection, known as immunoglobulins, constantly leak away in the urine. As a consequence, infection had been a common cause of death in the past. If these babies were to survive, they needed all the expertise of a children's hospital.

Holding the babies in my arms and examining them, I had no doubt that we should accept them for treatment. First, I needed to make the parents aware of the many risks involved in embarking on this course of action, and the limited chance of success. Weighed against supportive care alone, they agreed without exception to proceed. Initially, the battles we faced were against infection and in achieving adequate nutrition for the babies to stay safe and thrive. The dieticians devised a high calorie, high protein feeding regimen. Where it was poorly tolerated, supplemental night nasogastric tube feeds were employed. Eventually, we sought the help of a paediatrician who was expert in parenteral feeding, which is the delivery of liquid nutrition intravenously, through a line sited semi-permanently in a major blood vessel. Through this, we infused a concentrated albumin protein solution, derived from donated plasma, each night as the children slept. This and the special nutrition programme counteracted the urinary protein loss. It was a little like filling a sink with the plug half out of place but it proved successful. Against the odds, the babies thrived.

As the kidneys gradually deteriorated, urine production fell and the protein loss also tailed off. Dialysis was then necessary if we were to achieve the target weight. The children by now had their own personalities and each one became special to those of us involved in their treatment. When they became ill, we were desperate to see them recover. We struggled to appreciate how devastating it would be for their parents if we were to lose one. There was also an enormous sense of responsibility for undertaking an innovative treatment for the first time. The parents were an intrinsic part of the team and we felt almost part of the families. As such, we shared in their worries but had a responsibility to provide encouragement and allay their worst fears.

I started to plan for an eventual kidney transplant in such young children. It clearly needed to be performed in the children's hospital using all its facilities - the paediatric operating theatre and, post-operatively, the intensive care unit. A team from both renal units was assembled, including the transplant surgeon, senior theatre nurses, a paediatric surgeon and paediatric anaesthetists. We awaited suitable donated kidneys.

An unhelpful confrontation

Around this time, I sat down opposite a senior clinical administrator of the hospital group. I noted his pristine white coat and his tightly knotted club tie. He remained seated behind a mahogany desk.

"Thank you for finding the time to meet with me," he said with a smile, which I perceived as rather forced. It vanished quickly.

"Not at all, I was interested to find out why the administration of the adult hospital wished to see me, a paediatrician."

He picked up a pen and tapped it on an anonymous beige folder.

"Well, my answer to that is that I have certain responsibilities in relation to all three hospitals on the site. What happens in one can have knock-on effects in the others." His smile reappeared briefly.

"I see, but my understanding is that the Royal Belfast Hospital for Sick Children is more or less autonomous as the regional centre for paediatrics," I suggested.

"Mmm. Perhaps. What I actually wanted to discuss is that I understand you are performing dialysis on children in your unit?"

"Yes indeed. As you perhaps know, setting up such a provision was the reason for my appointment."

"That may be so, but I know of no funding having been received for such a development. Unfortunately, keen young chaps like yourself cannot just arrive and start spending money which does not exist."

Although I had red hair back then, I did not easily lose my temper but I was becoming extremely irritated by his negative attitude, which threatened everything I had been working for.

He continued, "I'm afraid you cannot go on with these plans. You will have to stop, until the service is properly costed and financed."

Having delivered this message, he started to rise from behind his desk, indicating our meeting was finished.

Astonished, I remained seated and, with an effort, spoke reasonably and calmly. Or so I hoped.

"First of all, there is an overall renal service budget which has been agreed with the chief executive of the Department of Health.It includes provision for paediatric nephrology. Can I suggest you have this discussion with him? Furthermore, the bulk of the expense for the dialysis materials we use is being borne by the City Hospital's renal unit, which supplies it, and with which I work closely. Indeed, we have been providing a dialysis and transplant programme based there for some time."

He had reluctantly retaken his seat and was no longer smiling.

"Secondly, you are correct, we are indeed supervising dialysis in three small children in our hospital, and finally, there is no question that I will stop their treatment, a course of action which would endanger their lives."

"I was merely making the point that you cannot continue to develop this service until the funding is secure."

He had perhaps begun to appreciate how incensed I had become, and that he was not in full command of the relevant facts.

"I doubt if you wish to speak with the parents yourself to deliver such news. I certainly will not be doing so."

I rose to my feet.

"I will of course report back the points you have raised regarding finances to our hospital manager, and to the renal unit administrator. I suggest you ask your finance department to liaise with them. I will, of course, alert them to the concerns you have raised. I expect you will be reassured that they are unfounded."

I left the office.

Improvising

Back in the intensive care unit, there was a more immediate problem. An infant admitted with severe sepsis had been on dialysis for 36 hours. He had been supportively anaesthetised and ventilated, in what is sometimes referred to as an induced coma. This was to protect his vital organs and give him the maximum chance of recovery. He required intravenous antibiotics and inotropic drugs to support his heart. At the most critical period of the illness, his blood pressure had fallen precipitously. As a result, his kidneys shut down. His cardiovascular status had since been stabilised and we expected the kidneys would slowly recover. However, the short-term problem with the impaired renal function was compounded by the volume of essential intravenous medication required to support his heart, to fight the infection and give him a chance of survival. His kidneys were no longer able to maintain an adequate urine output to balance the excess fluid involved. His heart was already stressed by the infection and an overload of fluids in his circulation might cause it to fail completely. The dialysis was addressing the imbalance by removing fluid and toxins.

Haemodialysis requiring a tiny artificial kidney and a machine safe to use for infants was not yet available. We were therefore dependent on peritoneal dialysis. A problem had developed with this, in that dialysis fluid had started to leak out around the temporary catheter where it passed through the child's thin abdominal wall. Apart from reducing the efficiency of the treatment, this was a potential source of infection and peritonitis. If fluid could leak out, bacteria might travel in.

I stopped the fluid cycles and drained the abdomen. I stitched a sterile, purse string suture around the catheter and closed the skin around it with a tight knot. A sample of the fluid was sent for bacterial culture. A few hours later the dialysis was restarted. Initially, there was no leak, but not for long.

I had a dilemma. If I removed the catheter and replaced it with another at a different position this would create two potential leak sites - and the current one might be difficult to seal. I reviewed whether it was necessary to continue dialysis with the intensive care specialists. The opinion was that, without it, the baby would inevitably deteriorate. I retired to my office with a cup of coffee to think.

A short time later, I climbed into my car and drove a mile or so to a nearby DIY store. I purchased two tubes of Superglue and returned to the intensive care unit. Like many people, I had accidentally stuck fingers together when using this substance and found it difficult to remove it with soap and water. I had heard a horror story from colleagues of a vengeful individual super-gluing the eyelids of an errant partner while they slept. I was thinking of trying it to seal the skin around the cannula.

I was not aware that field surgeons in the Vietnam war had used this type of glue to seal wounds, nor of its successful experimental use by plastic surgeons in Bradford, who had been overwhelmed by the need for multiple skin grafts for severe burns, after a recent football stadium fire.

I ensured the skin and tissues on the abdominal wall were completely dry, helped by the overhead heater which was maintaining the baby's temperature. I applied the superglue around the catheter. There was no obvious ill effect. It hoped it would bond rapidly but waited some minutes to be sure it had completely set.

The dialysis fluid was run back in and I intently watched the area around the cannula. There was no leak. Thirty minutes later we drained this fluid out and repeated the cycle. The skin remained dry. Success!

The superglue seal held for enough time to allow the baby's urine output to gradually increase over the next few days.

Inspiration

A gang of small children appeared charging around a street corner. They were right in the middle of the road. On a warm summer day, school was out, and they were in high spirits, shrieking and laughing as they came running and dancing down the hill. The bigger children at the front appeared to be pushing a supermarket trolley. At this speed, it was steering completely erratically.

Joanne, our Renal Nurse Specialist, was driving up the hill through the housing estate and watched the advancing horde, her eyes squinting in horror. Quickly she pulled over and brought her car to a halt as they hurtled towards her. She was on her way to visit a family who were managing a little girl on home dialysis. At that moment, she forgot her plan to assess how the parents were coping, and offer them advice and reassurance. She feared only that the metal trolley might crash into her precious little car. With hands clenched on the steering wheel, she cringed as it got closer.

At the last minute, the gang managed to swerve safely past.

But as they zoomed by, her eyes widened further and her mouth fell open. There was a small girl in the trolley. She held one hand aloft, pointing triumphantly onward, as the other gripped the side of her chariot.

It was her patient - one of the children with congenital nephrotic syndrome.

Deborah, for that was her name, was not up to running at the same speed as her friends. Her illness left her anaemic. It affected her size and muscle strength, but clearly not her spirit. She had commandeered transport, determined not to be left behind. Her face was alive, her blond hair flying in the wind.

Joanne breathed a sigh of relief and set off again. She was not long in the post, but extraordinary moments like this confirmed to her that she made the right move when transferring from the adult dialysis team. She became the lynchpin of our team. Deborah and she were destined to be lifelong friends.

Twenty-five years later, I stood beside her in a Batgirl outfit, on the rooftop of Belfast's Europa Hotel, once known as the most bombed hotel in Europe. I had been inveigled into wearing a Superman costume. Deborah grinned at me from behind her black mask and we were off, abseiling down the front wall. At the bottom she was ahead, as usual. This was a fundraising event for our local kidney research charity.

Five years after that day, I watched a video clip on a mobile phone. It showed her boyfriend getting down on one knee and asking for her hand in marriage.

Each of those first three babies with congenital nephrotic syndrome achieved the desired weight and size targets for dialysis and had successful kidney transplants.

Another battle

As the home programme grew, it became obvious that the families needed readily available practical support outside hospital. As ever, money for innovation was hard to find. The commissioning hierarchy had a problem employing a nurse, like Joanne, whose contracted work would, unconventionally, be as much in the community as in the hospital. Which area should bear the cost?

The British Kidney Patient Association came to the rescue. This national charity was set up by Mrs. Elizabeth Ward when her son developed kidney failure. Her aim was to provide practical, emotional and financial help to families, and to work with health professionals to improve health and care for renal patients. Hearing of the new service in Belfast, she suggested coming to visit.

"What is your greatest need at present?" she asked, after meeting the team and some of the patients.

The answer was, of course, for specialist staff to deliver training and home support. She proposed funding a post for two years in the first instance. Privately, she suggested that, in her experience, the hospital would have difficulty not absorbing the cost once the service was demonstrated to be essential. Her offer was accepted by management - but even then, we had to raise the nurse's travelling expenses from generous local donations, as these were not factored into the BKPA offer.

Learning to negotiate turned out to be a key part of my job. When dialysis machines were needed, it was sometimes easier to fall back on the generosity of the public and patient's relatives than to compete with other demands on the health service. Waiting in a queue to have new equipment requests considered could waste precious time. On occasions when purchases were made from charitable sources, thus saving the hospital money, there was often a reluctance by the administration to fund the contract for essential servicing costs. With time, these struggles became accepted as a routine part of running a service, although no less frustrating to fight. My early impatience and naivety about how the system worked developed into acceptance and a skill in anticipating problems and devising strategies in how to deal with bureaucracy.

Family support and rescue

I was fortunate that my family was enormously understanding about the demands of my job. We now had a third child, a little girl. Joanna was born in the maternity unit in which I trained as a student. In the labour ward, Anne was happy to allow a student midwife deliver our baby. An obstetrician friend stood by to talk the trainee through the correct procedure. I felt redundant, of course, and with Anne in control everything proceeded smoothly. When the crown of our baby's head became visible, the consultant calmly asked the nurse, "What must you do next?"

"Check there is no umbilical cord around the neck."

As she did so, I saw her eyes widen. She took a deep breath - whereas I stopped breathing.

"I *can* feel a loop of cord around the baby's neck!"

"What must you do now?"

"Loop the cord over the baby's head, away from the neck."

As he was saying, "go ahead", she was already doing it.

I started to breathe again.

Soon our little girl was in her mum's arms. She would become the athlete of the family.

Despite the demands of raising our children and her own jobs in nursing and medical research, Anne got to know many of my most ill patients. Once, she even prepared a favourite dinner for a girl who hated the hospital food and was refusing to eat. When I was worried or anxious, she always came to the rescue, willing to listen as I unburdened myself. I appreciated this support even more when a colleague told me his partner just did not want to hear anything about the hospital. Just being with my children, playing, reading bedtime stories, or later sharing in their worries, hopes, dreams and achievements was a therapy I possibly did not fully recognise back then. None of our three children developed an interest in following medicine as a career. Perhaps because we encouraged them to pursue their own interests, which they did with considerable success - but maybe, even subconsciously, they took note of all the ruined weekend and evening plans, when I was called away at the last minute.

My leave and holidays caused suspension of the "on call" status for the youngest patients. The adult nephrologists were willing to step in and cope with those of secondary school age if necessary, with care shared by my general paediatric colleagues. One, in particular, took a special interest in the renal patients. Dr Moira Stewart joined my Tuesday general renal clinic and became a favourite of many of the children. She was happy to hold the fort if I was temporarily unavailable. Eventually, I was delighted to have an excellent senior registrar, Dr Mary O'Connor, who developed an ambition of following in my footsteps.

I was loathe to abandon my general children's medicine work, but it was becoming inevitable, as the workload built. With support from fellow paediatricians and the adult team, a strong case for a second paediatric nephrologist was put forward to the Department of Health's review of all local Renal Services. The resulting report recommended this proposal be implemented and even supported, in time, the appointment of a third specialist. Dr O'Connor joined me after two years of nephrology higher specialist training in Bristol. At last I had a colleague, after managing single-handedly for 15 years. I soon recognised the special rapport she had with the children and families. A considerable weight eased from my shoulders. She already had significant experience of every aspect of our work. I valued her particular expertise in prescribing and supervising haemodialysis treatment, which we now performed regularly in a small three-bed unit. We were to spend many years happily working together.

16. Outpatient stories; needles, ghosts, and pennies

A new children's hospital?

With the renal replacement programme established at the children's hospital, the demands on my time inexorably increased. Since part of my salary was provided by the University, I had some responsibility for teaching paediatrics to medical students and co-ordinating research projects into hypertension and the genesis of coronary risk in childhood. Despite this, early in my consultant career, the Professor of Paediatrics suggested I take his place on the planning committee for a new, modern children's hospital. I protested that I was the most junior consultant.

"Exactly," he responded. "The chances of the project being completed during my tenure are slim, but there's a good chance you'll still be here to have the pleasure of working in the new hospital one day."

So I sat through many tortuous hours of meetings. Eventually, a minister of state, Lord Melchett committed £12 million for the project. Architects' plans and models were produced, modified, refined and … shelved. As I write this in retirement, there is still no new hospital and, sadly, Lord Melchett is no longer with us. The latest projected completion date is 2025.

Each week at my outpatient clinics, I had a real opportunity to get to know my patients. Learning of their family's background, circumstances, hopes and fears helped me understand how they were feeling and coping. Being the parent of a sick child is a frightening experience. To alleviate the emotional impact and win their trust, it was important to be attentive, empathetic, thoughtful and knowledgeable. A tall order.

In those 20-minute sessions, I also tried to grasp something of the children's personalities. I wanted to understand how the illness and worries upset their daily lives and schooling. Inevitably, they had been warned to be on their best behaviour in front of the doctor. Waiting is not something small children do well and clinics could run late. I was once horrified to overhear a bored, rowdy child being threatened by their mother.

229

"If you do not settle down and behave, I will get the doctor to give you an injection."

So, I attempted to break down the image of the big scary doctor by chatting directly to each child, and treating them the way I did my own children, or my nieces and nephews. I explored what interested them and stored the information for future visits. I tried to answer honestly any questions they had. Parents, already on edge, sometimes worried that a child was being too outspoken or rude in these exchanges but I relished their lack of inhibition, because it meant I could grasp some understanding of the way they were thinking. I regarded success as being treated by them as an equal, or even as a grown-up friend.

Memories of busy sessions tend to focus on the more dramatic encounters.

No needles Norman

Norman entered a couple of paces behind his mum, head down, dragging his schoolbag and his feet. I assessed the scene.

"Hi Norman, I see your team scraped a win on Saturday."

"What do you mean, scraped a win? Spurs are rubbish, they couldn't score a goal if the net was a mile wide."

He had straightened up; his chin jutted out a little. Remembering which football team or sport a child supports is an important part of being a children's doctor. There is more than one way of breaking through a defence.

He looked at a pile of Lego pieces and sat down on the floor beside it.

His mum allowed herself a slight smile as she burrowed into her handbag. She withdrew a notebook. In it she kept a record of the results of the daily tests she performed on her son's urine. She informed me that protein had been showing up for a week, but she had not contacted me, as she had already got that day's appointment in her diary.

Norman had a relapsing and remitting form of nephrotic syndrome, a variety of the condition which usually has a good ultimate outcome. When it flares up, proteins leak through the kidney filter into the urine. If this is not detected early enough, a patient will become unwell and retain fluid, often first revealed by puffy eyes and swollen legs.

While we reviewed her record, Norman seemed disinterested, and was attempting to assemble a giant tower of Lego bricks.

"What is protein anyway?" said a small voice from the floor.

What could I tell an eight-year-old?

"Does your mum ever make jelly?" I asked.

"Mmm. I love jelly. We had jelly trifle on my birthday."

"Do you know how she makes it?"

He set down the bricks, put a finger to his mouth and closed his eyes.

"She boils a kettle of water and pours some into a bowl, gets a packet of jelly powder stuff, puts it into the bowl, stirs them together and it all turns red."

"They're called jelly crystals." His mum interjected, giving me a curious look.

"Then what?"

"She puts the bowl in the fridge and when she takes it out again, Abracadabra, the water has turned into jelly." Pleased, he held his chin out again.

"Well, proteins are a bit like jelly crystals, making blood thicker than water.Do you remember your legs got really fat when you first came to hospital and it slowed you up playing football? That was water swelling your legs, because there was not enough protein in your blood. We gave you medicine to build your protein back up which thickened your blood and drew the water back out of your ankles."

Dubious, he rolled his eyes, and returned to the Lego. This explanation would not have satisfied a scientist, nor it seemed, Norman. I turned back to his mother.

"Your record suggests we are early in a relapse and it is possible the protein will disappear again spontaneously. Sometimes a head cold can trigger a relapse and as it resolves so does the protein leak. If not, he will need a course of steroid tablets."

"I really hope that will not be necessary. I know the steroids work, but you know how they have upset him in the past."

I agreed steroid treatment could have an unfortunate effect on children's behaviour. I was thinking of one younger boy who was nearly banned from his nursery school for aggressive behaviour. He had bitten several other kids in squabbles over toys. Norman's mother spoke again.

"I know Norman is quite a sensible lad nowadays, and I'm sure he will manage better as he gets older. It's just that the tablets made him so hyper the last time he was on them. He never seemed to sit still, and we had trouble getting him over to sleep at night."

I suggested quietly that we did a blood test to determine how far his plasma protein level had fallen so we could decide whether it was possible to hold off the treatment for a week or so. That was, if she was prepared to take the risk of a full relapse while we awaited the result - which could then mean a longer course of tablets to reverse the effects.

"Okay," she said, her voice dropping to a whisper, "but we'll need to talk him into agreeing. The first thing he said when we got here today was, 'no needles'."

I also found myself dropping my voice.

"I'll ask the nurse to put some anaesthetic cream on his arm to numb the skin, so the needle doesn't hurt him."

We turned to explain the plan to Norman and found ourselves looking at an abandoned pile of Lego bricks.

I pulled the curtain back from around the examination couch. His mum looked underneath the couch, all that was there was a school backpack. We realised my clinic door was slightly open.

"My God, he's done a runner!" she exclaimed as she rushed into the waiting area.

"Did a little boy with fair hair in a blue school uniform run out?" She called to the other waiting parents. The clerk looked up from her desk and put her hand to her mouth.

"I thought he was just hurrying to catch up with his mum."

Norman's mother was already dashing across the foyer. We phoned the security office to ask that they try to intercept him.

Twenty minutes later Norman was marched back in.

"I caught him at the end of the hospital road, near the front gates," said his mum, still catching her breath. "It must be nearly half a mile away. I'm knackered from running after him. I'm so embarrassed. There will be no jelly for this boy for a long time."

"There's no need to apologise. Look on the positive side. You have a strong, fit lad with plenty of spirit, despite his bouts of illness. We are used to dealing with kids who hate needles. It's only to be expected. One of my colleagues has a patient whose mum calls her 'No Veins Jane', because the doctors and nurses have great trouble finding one to take a sample."

I turned to her son.

"Nobody likes a blood test, Norman. Do you think you could help me this time and point out which of your veins you reckon would be the best one to use?"

I wrapped a tourniquet around his upper arm as I talked.

"You probably remember the spray we sometimes use to freeze your skin? It's the same stuff football coaches use on players who injure their leg. If you pick a vein, you could freeze your arm for me. That way you can be sure the needle won't hurt."

Reluctantly, he pointed at a plumped up vein in the crook of this left elbow. I handed him the aerosol canister. He spayed an excessive amount of alcohol onto his arm. I slipped the needle in and in seconds it was all over and I was placing a sticking plaster on the puncture site.

"Brilliant work, Norman, maybe I could give you a job doing this."

"Wise up!" he responded, his pride restored.

"Actually, I think I'd rather have one quick needle prick than the pain from a kick in the shins at football." I said.

I could just make out a conciliatory mumble in reply. "I bet you wear shin pads."

The ghost story

"Hello, Aisling. Good morning, Mrs. Norris. I hope the traffic wasn't too bad on the long trip to get here."

Aisling made no response, slumping into a chair with her fair hair falling across her face as she looked down at her hands. I looked at her mum and raised my eyebrows quizzically. She briefly rolled her eyes and gave an almost imperceptible shake of her head.

"Any problems with the dialysis?" I asked. "I gather that Joanne, our nurse, thinks you're coping very well."

"Yes, yes, we are. It's not the dialysis, doctor," said Aisling's mum, twisting the ring on her finger.

"It is something else," she added quietly."Something that Aisling doesn't want to talk about."

I turned to Aisling.

"Is there anything I can do to help?"

She shook her head.

I let the matter drop, hoping all was well at home. There is an inevitable strain placed on families by the responsibility of three or four CAPD bag changes each day, keeping records, carefully dispensing medicines, and providing a special diet. All these drained time away from the normal daily routine - especially for other children in the household.

I examined Aisling, checking her blood pressure and taking a blood sample for testing. Then I suggested that she went off with Joanne to have her catheter exit site checked in the clinical room next door.

My expression signalled to Joanne that maybe she could suss out the problem. She rested a friendly hand on the girl's waist as she guided her out.

The door closed.

"It's not the treatment doctor. We've all got used to everything involved-in the home dialysis and up until Aisling started back at secondary school, she seemed so much better. Her appetite improved, and she had more energy. She was back going about with her friends at weekends, then over a few weeks she became more withdrawn. We have tried to find out what is upsetting her, but she ends up getting cross, and tells us just to leave her alone."

I knew Aisling as a pleasant, quiet, shy girl. Defeated, I moved on to talk of more straightforward matters - fluid balance and blood results. These showed she remained relatively anaemic but not to a degree that warranted

234

blood transfusion, with its concurrent risks. For renal patients these include the possibility of sensitisation to foreign tissue types, thus increasing the possibility of subsequent rejection of a donor kidney. The anaemia is due to a failure of the normal kidney production of Erythropoietin, or Epo, a hormone which stimulates bone marrow to generate red blood cells. It would be some years before synthetic Epo became available, dramatically improving patient's lives - and, coincidently, illegally enhancing the performance of certain professional cyclists and athletes.

When the family had left, Joanne reappeared, held both her hands out, palms upwards, towards me, then clenched them into fists and grimaced. She had discovered that Aisling was being bullied at school. Some kids had nicknamed her Ghosty and had been taunting her. With her fair hair, she had natural pale skin and now her anaemia exaggerated the pallor. Joanne didn't know how this all started. Aisling was a pretty girl and she speculated that perhaps some boy who fancied her but got no encouragement had turned nasty. The bullies, having invented the nickname, realised this upset Aisling, then ganged up on her in school, chanting the name and calling it out from hiding places.

She stopped and muttered under her breath, "The little cowards! As if she hasn't got enough to contend with."

At the next nurse home visit, a suggestion was made to Mrs. Norris, that we discreetly contact the school, and this was agreed. The dialysis home care nurse spoke with the head teacher, explaining she wanted to discuss a matter concerning a pupil in strictest confidence - with her mother's permission. He listened carefully to the story and clearly knew exactly which pupil Joanne was talking about. It was emphasised that Aisling would be mortified if she thought she'd broken the golden rule of never telling tales or being a snitch. He was sympathetic and promised to do his best to sort out the problem. He inquired when exactly she would next be at the clinic.

Later, we learnt that he called a meeting of the year group while Aisling was absent. We never knew what exactly was said but it was undoubtedly made clear that the school would not tolerate pupils who bullied others. As well as physical intimidation, we gathered that he specifically mentioned using cruel nicknames to make people's time at school miserable.

No victims or antagonists were named - but the culprits must have recognised the headmaster's threats were aimed at them. Perhaps they believed he knew their identity, perhaps they felt guilty. His talk initially had considerable effect.

I knew nothing of this when Aisling returned to the clinic over the next month or two, but I noticed the return of her old, shy smile. Years later, I learned from her that there were other unpleasant nicknames used by the same nasty pupils and she was relieved when at last she was able to finish with school.

The bullies perhaps did more harm than her illness - but the name-calling eventually became irrelevant when a successful transplant transformed her life and complexion.

The swimmer

On the day before her clinic appointment, Lucy skipped to the water's edge, looked down, a smile of anticipation on her face. She raised her hands above her head, fingertips touching, closed her eyes, took a deep breath and dived. Surfacing, she flicked long hair away from her face, broke into a smooth front crawl, hardly creating a ripple as she pulled away. Twenty minutes later she emerged and wrapped herself in a large fluffy towel before getting dry and dressed. She headed for home, reinvigorated, bouncing from foot to foot.

Next morning, she was at the hospital for her regular check-up. She greeted Brid, today's dialysis nurse, with a hug and held out an arm for the blood pressure cuff. She watched as the skin over her forearm was cleaned with an alcohol wipe and winced as a needle was slipped into her vein for a blood sample. She chatted away, mentioning her previous day's swim to take her mind off the sharp zing of the puncture. Brid frowned as she reached for a plaster and talked to Lucy quietly and seriously.

They moved through the adjoining door into the doctor's room. I was sitting alongside the desk. Lucy plumped herself down in the chair opposite me. I looked up with a welcoming smile, but before I could speak, she said, "Brid has just told me you don't approve of your patients going swimming?"

I looked at her, curious. My eyes narrowed as I tried to be diplomatic,

236

"Not completely. It's the risk of contamination and infection around the exit site where the dialysis tube enters the tummy. If germs travel down the track it can lead to peritonitis which is dangerous and painful."

"I'm a keen swimmer, always have been," she continued in an exhibition of adolescent selective deafness and nonchalance. "I love to get into the water at this time of year."

"Most people are actually too self-conscious to swim because of the tube; it creates a noticeable bulge under tight swimsuits," I pointed out, hoping to deflect her from her choice of sport, rather than spoil her enthusiasm for exercise. "It's not so obvious under a loose T shirt," I added.

Brid was standing by the examination couch. "Let's have a look at the exit site."

"There is no one around to see me when I swim."

I failed to hide my concern and asked if she had access to a private pool.

"No, I'm a country girl, you know. I swim in a little lake near our farm."

The nurse and doctor exchanged wide-eyed looks out of Lucy's line of sight. We were both thinking of things like cow dung, wild animal excreta, and rat urine and how they propagated Leptospirosis infection.

Brid peeled back the dressings which had been applied meticulously around the tube and over it. The exit site was spotless except for some yellow skin discolouration caused by iodine antiseptic solution. She sighed with relief.

Lucy grinned.

I shrugged and shook my head in defeat. Then my face brightened with an idea.

"Brid, do you think there are any of those clear adherent waterproof wound dressings or maybe a stoma bag in our Theatre?"

She returned shortly with a selection.

"You know, one of these applied over the normal dressings might be just the thing for our mermaid."

A special Christmas present

On a dull, cold winter day, the door opened and a pretty blonde-haired girl bounced in ahead of her sister and mother. The gloom lifted.

"Well, did you girls get everything you wanted from Santa?"

Rebecca's eyes sparkled as she rattled off a list before her sister could respond. At the top was the latest pink Barbie doll. She was a real girly-girl.

"I bet the two of you got some nice things to wear, too."

The younger girl had been listening tolerantly but now got a chance to give a few details of the toys she found under the Christmas tree.

"Pink is my sister's favourite colour," she added, something I already knew from our regular meetings over several years.

My examination completed, and her blood pressure checked. I reviewed her recent test results and progress with their mother. My conclusion was that Rebecca had had an excellent spell and, as I made some notes, I expressed the hope that this would be a really good year for her. I predicted that she would be fine and healthy in the long run.

"Do you know what dad got mummy for Christmas?".

I looked up. My patient was sitting with her elbows on my desk, waiting for my reply. I thought I detected a mischievous glint in the eyes she had fixed on me..

"Actually, I don't.".

I turned towards her mum. A flicker of anxiety crossed her face. She reached a hand out, in an attempt to silence her daughter. She was too late..

"He got her a lovely red silk nightie with soft white fur around the edges," she announced, evading her mother's grip.

The two girls shrieked with laughter. Their mum's face was now probably the same colour as the nightie.

"Girls, girls! The doctor doesn't need to know everything."

She chased them, still giggling, out through the door.

Find a penny, pick it up

While reviewing a little girl who had been admitted with a severe attack of asthma a few weeks earlier, I inquired how she had been faring, and whether she had experienced any shortness of breath when she was playing or running, I was distracted by the noisy breathing of a younger child, who was sitting beside us in a buggy. Concentrating on the task at hand, I warmed my stethoscope, placed it on my patient's chest and listened. I was pleased that there was no wheeze to be heard. Removing it from my ears, I was again aware of a crowing sound coming from the toddler. I checked my patient's ability to use the inhalers I'd prescribed to control her symptoms. She took pride in demonstrating how good her technique was. I showed her a device which could measure how hard she could blow - and suggested competing with her mum to see who could blow the marker to the highest number on the scale. Her peak expiratory flow rate was excellent, as was her mother's. As she had another go, I told her mum I was really pleased with her response to treatment.

"Before you go, can I just ask about her brother's noisy breathing?" I asked. "Have you had him checked by your family doctor?"

"Yes," she replied. "He said he had a croup caused by a virus and it should gradually settle."

"Do you mind if I ask how long he's had it?"

She thought for a minute.

"Since before his sister came into hospital, so maybe three weeks or more. I haven't worried about it as it doesn't bother Jake, and hopefully it will clear up soon. Do you think he has a bit of asthma, too?"

"May I have a quick listen to his chest, just to check?"

She removed his coat and top gently. I noticed that the little hollow above his breastbone at the base of his throat was sucked inwards each time he inhaled, with an accompanying croaky stridor. There was also a softer noise when he breathed out. I listened and concluded the sound was coming from his upper airway, not from deep in his chest. I knew that croup, which comes from inflammation and narrowing of the windpipe and larynx, is short-lived.

"This little man's chest is clear, but the croup generally resolves in days and does not persist for a month. I'd like to get a quick X-ray if you wouldn't mind?"

"Oh doctor, are you sure he needs it? You don't think it could be anything serious, do you?"

She was already searching for a tissue in her handbag.

"No, no, I don't think so. It's just a precaution because it has persisted. I agree he seems perfectly healthy, but I would be happier to get a picture while you are here, just to check his windpipe hasn't becomea little narrowed."

I patted her hand and stepped out to speak quickly with a staff nurse, explaining I had worried the mum. I asked the nurse to stay with her while the picture was taken and to bring the film back to me.

Fifteen minutes later my phone rang. It was the radiologist.

"I am sending round the X-ray but wanted to warn you first. I've never seen this before, but there is what looks like a penny coin resting vertically at the larynx. If it were to flip over it could block the whole airway."

I had not expected this. I put the film up on the light box and pointed out the coin to the mother. She was understandably shocked.

"He is safe for now, if the coin stays where it is, but we need to get it out as soon as possible. I want to admit him and get the ear, nose and throat specialist to see him today."

The nurse took over again, helping the worried mother phone her husband and the children's grandparents, while I contacted the ENT surgeon on call.

By late afternoon, the penny was in a small specimen bottle, following a skilful extraction using a bronchoscope. I was glad I did not have to administer any anaesthetic for this delicate procedure.

Jake was sitting on his dad's knee, breathing quietly and playing happily with a new toy. His mum knelt in front of him smiling. Next day he was off home.

17. Disturbing phone calls

Christmas confusion

On Boxing Day each year, my brother, a church minister, and his wife hosted an annual family gathering. All afternoon and evening, their house would be noisy and full with at least eight adults, plus children and grandchildren. When everyone had long gone and the manse was at last quiet, with the dishes washed and the debris cleared, the hosts would collapse into the cocoon of a warm bed. Ron liked to relive the good-natured banter of sibling rivalry rekindled during the day's party games, as he drifted into a contented sleep.

One year, in the early hours of the morning, his slumber was shattered by the shrill ringing of the bedside phone. He jumped up to silence the noise which had wrecked his dreams. Who could be calling at this hour? Had some tragedy or death befallen a relative or parishioner? He held the handset against his ear.

"Hello, I apologise for disturbing you. Am I speaking to Doctor Savage?"

Still coming fully awake, he confirmed this. He held a doctorate in divinity from Princeton University.

"Thank you, doctor, this is the UK Transplant Service. We have a donated kidney which I would like to offer you, as it seems an excellent match for one of your patients."

The Reverend Savage was now sitting upright in bed, his wife watching anxiously as he stammered uncharacteristically.

"I'm afraid there has been some sort of mistake. I think it is my brother you need to speak to, not me. How did you get my number?"

"It was passed on to me by the nurse in charge of the Children's renal unit just now."

"Ah! Their Dr Savage is my brother. He has been visiting us this afternoon and evening past, but returned home several hours ago. I can give you his home number."

As I was on standby to receive any organ offers that morning, I had given the staff the number at which I might be contacted for the rest of the day. It had been written on a card, and taped to the console above the ward phone, but with no indication that it was only to be tried if there was no response from my home number.

Ron enjoyed recounting this story - and it may even have been used on occasion to illustrate one of his sermons.

Phone allergy

Over the years, I developed a sort of emotional allergic reaction to the noise of our home phone. Any time the phone rang between 10 p.m. and 7 a.m., I instantly awoke with my resting heart rate doubling within seconds. Would it be a transplant offer, or a dialysis problem? The spectre of peritonitis always sprang to mind.

The efficiency of peritoneal dialysis is time limited, with any episode of peritonitis likely to compromise the permeability and filtering efficiency of the peritoneal membrane. To avoid this, rapid antibiotic treatment is essential, no matter what hour of the day or night it is suspected. In time, we had moved to employ automated PD cycling machines with sophisticated alarm systems. Since they delivered overnight treatment while children slept, any worries or problems were most likely to be reported outside normal working hours. Parents and patients were trained to immediately make contact if there was any abdominal discomfort or if the drained fluid looked cloudy. If they did so, it was almost guaranteed that they and I would quickly be en route to the hospital.

At home, we subscribed to the then-novel "call waiting" service on the house landline, so that my children would hang up if they were alerted to another incoming call.

For a time, a local taxi service had a number only two digits different from our private one. Occasionally, in the early hours of the morning, an inebriated customer would call to demand a cab at some city night spot. Although tempted to agree and hang up, I merely advised them to contact the correct number and quickly returned to sleep. Anne, irritated by these calls, sometimes had more trouble getting back to sleep, and later demanded

242

to know how I was able to do so. I explained, "If it is not the hospital, I am so relieved, I relax and drift off."

Actually, I was more likely to have sleep ruined by a junior doctor whose opening words were invariably, "I'm phoning just to let you know," before expanding on some clinical diagnosis or decision they had made. I detested this phrase and lay awake wondering if they'd been hoping I would offer to go into the hospital and confirm their approach was correct? If not, why phone at all? Was it just so that they could say they had consulted with me in the awful eventuality that something went wrong? Depending on my knowledge of the person, I may have been compelled to drag myself out of bed and drive to the hospital to make sure everything was well before I could settle again. Worse still was a rare, discreet, follow-up call from an experienced nurse, suggesting it might be good if I did arrive, while swearing me to secrecy about her action.

Florida

Disturbing calls sometimes came from patients on holiday abroad.

"Hello doctor. Thank goodness I was able to reach you. The thing is, some friends we've made here offered to take Simon water skiing on the lake. He's never had the chance to try this before and it seemed too good an opportunity to miss. He managed quite well and had great fun, although he fell into the water a few times. We were glad when he returned safely to the dock. That was when we discovered the protective cap on his PD line had become disconnected. It's gone! Lake water may have gone down the tube."

The mother paused for a breath.

"Just remind me of where you are holidaying," I interjected. "I think it's in Florida and we identified a contact dialysis centre nearby for you. Is that correct?"

"What should we do? Should we go there? Will they know what to do?"

Her voice was rising, tears were not far away.

"This is not the first time a cap has been dislodged. The centre has a letter which we sent to them, giving all Simon's medical details. You have a copy, too. There's no need to panic, just take him along. They will give him antibiotics and a new cap and perhaps renew the line. Bring all your insurance documents with you, if possible."

I was wondering how polluted the lake might be.

Simon's father came on the line.

"All the paperwork is back in the hotel, but I drove past the medical centre a few days ago. It is only a few miles away, so I think I can find it again. I'm suggesting we just go there straight away and worry about the paperwork later."

A listening nurse slid Simon's clinical notes across my desk.

"I can give you the address again if you need it. Do you have a pen? When you get there ask for Dr Julian Ullrich. He is the nephrologist we corresponded with. I am sure he will be able to sort everything out. How is the boy? Do you want me to have a word with him?"

"He seems absolutely fine. Quite unconcerned, but not amused that he has to go to hospital and will not be allowed to go water skiing again. Maybe the less fuss the better, doc."

I read out the address and wished them good luck.

The line went dead.

I reflected on this story when I was contacted about a similar problem some time later. No foreign lake was involved this time, just soapy bath water. A three-year-old managed to unscrew the cap from his dialysis catheter when his mother's back was turned, searching for shampoo. He was quickly hoisted out of the bath and a new cap connected. Neither boy came to any harm when the residual fluid in the abdomen was drained out and antibiotic treatment instituted.

Torremolinos

When the blood chemistry is no longer satisfactorily controlled by peritoneal dialysis and no donor kidney is yet available, haemodialysis becomes the next option. First, an arteriovenous fistula is created in the forearm. This involves vascular surgery, in which an artery is attached to an adjacent vein. Some of the arterial blood flow, going towards the hand, is short circuited into the vein which expands and dilates. Needles can then be inserted relatively easily into the visibly-swollen vessel. Blood is drawn through the needle into the kidney machine and pumped through an artificial kidney, before being returned to the circulation. Understandably, some children are distressed by the needling procedure, despite the use of local anaesthetic on the skin and even light sedation. Not surprisingly an occasional child develops a sort of needle phobia. Their anxiety and fear of the treatment can dominate their life. An alternative is to place a double lumen venous catheter into a large vessel, usually the subclavian vein which drains the arm vessels and then runs under the collar bone, or clavicle. This tube is connected directly to the haemodialysis machine, thus overcoming any needle phobia. Blood is drawn from one lumen and returned through the other. The catheters are held in place by a cuff on the tubing which secures it under the skin, and further anchored by adhesive dressings.

Eventually, a choice between all dialysis modalities was offered to all new patients.

On a summer morning, a call came through to the ward from a family holidaying in Torremolinos on the Spanish coast. "Dr Savage, Megan's central line has been pulled right out during some boisterous play in the hotel swimming pool."

I could just make out the message above the background noise of excited children and booming music. I was thinking, "Oh my God," but managed not to verbalise my reaction.

"Has she lost much blood? Is she still bleeding?"

Thankfully, her mother could hear me clearly.

"No, there isn't a spot of blood to be seen or I wouldn't be so calm. What should we do?"

"You need to get her to the hospital where she's been having her haemodialysis. In the meantime, get some sterile gauze from the dressing packs we gave you to take with you. Press it firmly over the exit site until you get there. Can you look carefully at the surrounding skin and tell me if there's any swelling?"

"There is nothing to see, just the small hole where the catheter came out. No bulge and no blood."

"Great, we are going to be okay then. Phone the hospital and tell them you are on your way, and why. Can you get the other kids looked after and drive there? If not, ask the hospital or the hotel to get an ambulance."

She assured that all the family could squeeze into a hire car.

"Remember, keep some pressure on the site. Let me know what happens. Don't waste any time. Go!"

That evening, the Spanish unit confirmed there had been no significant blood loss. They had elected not to attempt to replace the catheter. They had noticed the fistula which Megan had vehemently refused to let us use some months earlier, because of her fear of needles. Amazingly, they had persuaded her to have a haemodialysis session using a relatively large needle inserted into the fistula. The staff played to her vanity, telling her how lovely she looks with her Spanish suntan as they slipped it into her arm. She had several more sessions before returning home. Her parents were justly proud of her.

"Those Torremolinos nurses are really brilliant," she told our nurses, tactlessly. She did, however, allow them to continue using the fistula.

A borrowed car

On a quiet Saturday afternoon, the house was still and it was warm enough to sit outside with a cup of coffee and the newspaper. My eyes were closing in the sun when I heard the phone in the distance. Reluctantly, I walked back inside, picked it up, and immediately recognised the voice as the mother of one of my renal patients.

"I've never called you at home before, and I apologise, but Daniel has just given us a real scare. He had some sort of turn; he started to shiver and shake, and he looked as if he was out of it for a minute. He seems to be all right now. We are going to bring him to the emergency department but wondered if you might be able to see him there."

This family had a number of bad scares when their boy was critically ill and, although he was fully recovered, I understood their concern. They lived quite close to my home, so I could be with them in a few minutes.

"Stay where you are. I'll come up to your house first. What number is it? I can be with you more quickly than you can get to the hospital."

I grabbed my medical bag and searched the hall table for our car keys. They were nowhere to be seen. I kicked the table, and, mentally, myself. Of course! Anne had gone shopping in the family car. How could I be so stupid. I considered using my bicycle, although the route finished straight up an extremely steep hill.

Then I noticed a single door key on the table. It was the key to our friend's house across the road. They had left it with us when they went off on holiday.

Their second car was in the driveway and I was fairly sure I knew where their keys were kept hidden. I ran to their front door, entered the hall, opened the concealed door of a cupboard hidden under the stairs and felt inside. Yes, the car keys were there! I dashed out of the house and unlocked the old car. It started first time.

I drove fast, probably breaking the speed limit, ignoring the fact that I was unlikely to be insured and, technically, was in charge of a stolen vehicle.

I safely arrived at Daniel's home. He was bright and alert. He did not have a temperature. His blood pressure was fine. A quick neurological and cardiac examination gave normal results. I reassured the parents, then phoned my registrar to arrange for Daniel to be admitted for some tests and 24 hours observation. I left, promising to call and see them and review the results a little later. I didn't tell them then that I did not want to chance driving across the city until I could do so in my own car. Daniel's tests were fine and he remained well.

The broken leg

A phone call was put through to my room just before the Monday clinic started.

"Doctor, I apologise for bothering you, but I wondered if it would be possible for you to see Martin today? He doesn't have an appointment but he broke his leg playing rugby on Saturday."

I was immediately concerned, as Martin had recently finished an eight-week course of steroids.

"Of course, where is he at the minute?"

"Oh, he is at school, I don't like him to miss any more days than necessary. I will be collecting him shortly."

This news caused me some relief. Martin had recently completed a short course of Prednisolone, a powerful steroid, to terminate a relapse of his kidney condition. These drugs must be used judiciously because of their potential side effects. In the case of children's bones, growth may be delayed by long courses, and osteoporosis can result from its use, with an associated reduction in bone density and strength. Despite this possibility, I had given the go-ahead for him to return to contact sport once he was well and off medication.

Having agreed to add the boy to my list of patients that morning, I requested that his clinical notes were pulled and brought to me. Before he arrived, I checked his recent blood tests. His biochemical bone profile, calcium and phosphate levels were normal, as were his bone enzymes. A routine bone scan had shown no evidence of osteoporosis. On that basis I had explained to his mother that I thought there was little risk in a 12-year-old playing rugby - as long as the school was aware of his medical background. He had been provided with a card stating any current and previous steroid treatment.

Martin hobbled in on two crutches, with his lower left leg encased in plaster.

"I'm really sorry to hear about your accident, I'm sure it was quite painful."

"It wasn't too bad and it's ok now, except for having to use crutches."

"How did it happen exactly? A tackle, a scrum? Or did the leg just give way?" I hoped it wasn't the latter.

"No, actually it was the schoolteacher's fault,"

"The schoolteacher? Really? How come?"

"Yes, he was refereeing when he tripped and fell on top of me. He's a big heavy man, about six foot tall. The rest of the boys thought it was hilarious, until they realised I really couldn't walk."

His mother spoke up.

"I didn't think it was funny when the school phoned to say he was on his way to the accident and emergency department at our local hospital. I was worried sick because of the steroid tablets he was on a few months ago. The doctors there reassured me there was nothing to worry about, as it was only the small bone in his leg, the fibula I think it's called, which was broken, and the ends were still closely aligned. They seemed to be sure it would heal all right, but I wanted to check with you."

I confirmed that they were probably correct, although it might take a little longer than usual.

"All Martin is worried about is that he's lost his place on the team," she concluded.

I sympathised with him and offered some positive news.

"Martin, in the clinic along the corridor, is an orthopaedic surgeon, a bone doctor. He is also a top rugby referee. I am going to get him to keep an eye on you. He may want to take a few X-rays of your leg over the next few weeks to see how quickly it is healing. He's also quite expert in sports injuries and can help you get back to full fitness in the shortest time. How does that sound?"

I called Harry, my colleague, and a much happier Daniel headed off to see him.

What's next, I wondered?

Motorbike madness

"Doctor, when we started Peter's peritoneal dialysis tonight, we immediately noticed that the fluid that drained out was quite red. We think there is blood in it."

"Does he seem unwell? Does he have a temperature? Is he in pain? Is his tummy tender to touch?"

"No, none of those things, but I should tell you he was in a junior Motocross competition today. I don't think you know that he has a small scrambler motorbike. The race was in a field on a rough track-with several mounds. Coming off a jump from one of these, he was thrown off, into the soft mud, and the next rider drove over him. He seemed unhurt and jumped back on the bike and managed to finish third!"

Indeed, I had no idea Peter was into motorbikes. I advised that he be brought in so I could check him over. We met up in the ward a short time later. I found nothing significant - but we ran several quick cycles of dialysis fluid into his abdomen, almost immediately draining it out again. By the third exchange, the fluid was crystal clear, with no discolouration. I sent some off for analysis and bacteriological culture.

Peter was nonchalant as we carried out an abdominal X-ray and scan. They were normal. We kept him in overnight for observation during completion of his usual night-time dialysis program. He remained pain free and the fluid stayed clear. As a precaution, I introduced some prophylactic antibiotics into the last fluid cycle. The antibiotic would remain in his abdomen for the next 12 hours until he went back on the automated PD machine as usual in the evening. This overnight routine left him free of treatment by day, and in his case free to take part in motorbike sports. The sort of a problem he had presented to me was not covered in standard dialysis or nephrology textbooks

Taking risks on a motorbike proved that illness did not completely control Peter's life. He was discharged home unharmed.

Thirty years later I believe he is still a biker.

A French conversation

The family of one of our patients decided to spend a holiday in a static caravan at a campsite in the Vendée region of France. Their daughter required haemodialysis three times a week. They asked if we could arrange for her to be treated in a French unit while they were there.

I knew there was a reciprocal arrangement between the French Health Service and the NHS but I blanched at the thought of setting this up.

"How is your French?" I enquired. They made non-committal noises then volunteered, "Jill is learning it at school. We hope the holiday will help with that."

Jill was 12 years old.

"Where exactly will you be staying?" I asked, with a sinking heart.

"Pornic on the Atlantic coast. Do you know it?"

By chance I did - and I also knew there was a regional paediatric renal unit in Nantes some 50 kilometres away. I had met the senior nephrologist there at European research meetings. He presented his work at these events in fluent English.

I agreed to attempt to get in touch with him over the next few days. I located the hospital phone number in the European Society for Paediatric Nephrology (ESPN) membership handbook.

In preparation for the call, I sketched out a few key phrases I might use, reflecting that I had only scraped through French exams in my youth.

"Bonjour madame. Je voudrais parler au Docteur Cochat, s'il vous plaît".

I spoke in my best schoolboy French. The switchboard operator in Nantes replied in a rapid, and to me incomprehensible, flurry of consonants. Fortunately, this was followed by a series of beeps and a ringing tone.

"Bonjour. Docteur Cochat ici, comment puis-je vous aider?"

"Bonjour Pierre, I hope you do not mind me speaking in English. I am Docteur Maurice Savage, a nephrologist in Ireland. You may not remember me, but we have met at ESPN meetings." There was a moment's silence, so I continued.

"I have a favour to ask. I have a child who will be holidaying near Nantes in the summer, and I wished to discuss the possibility of her receiving haemodialysis in your unit."

There was a longer pause.

"Mais, je suis un psychiatre. I am a psychiatrist. Je pense que vous voulez parler avec mon collègue Pierre."

Words failed me, especially French words. There were apparently two doctor Cochats.

I stuttered.

"Merci monsieur. Je m'excuse. Au revoir."

I hung up embarrassed and nonplussed. I sat looking at the phone. I would have to start all over. Would I end up babbling incoherently to the psychiatrist again? My nursing friends who had been listening found my discomfort amusing.

Then, a brainwave. Michael, the father of one of my patients, taught French at a local school. I contacted him and explained my difficulty. He was happy to help. A few days later, he arrived to collect his son after his dialysis session. I had noted down some of Jill's details for him. He phoned the hospital for me, easily got through to the correct department, explained he was calling on my behalf, omitting to explain why. Then he handed me the phone, smiling.

"Maurice, mon ami." said a voice at the other end. "Of course, we will be happy to accommodate your patient."

18. Difficult questions

Small children often ask quite unexpected questions. Finding the right answer can challenge the most able paediatrician, but they help to keep us grounded.

"Why are veins blue, Doctor Savage?"

"It's to do with the amount of oxygen in the blood, I think," I suggested to a seven-year-old. I knew this explanation was going right over his head. He ignored me.

"Yes, but when you take some blood from the vein in my arm, it's always red, not blue."

"It's difficult to explain."

I'm rescued by his mother.

"Stop pestering the doctor and be quiet."

I smiled my gratitude while thinking, 'Why *are* veins blue?'

"Will you change my nappy?" A toddler stepped in front of me and looked up at my face, interrupting the ward round.

The nurses and junior doctor grinned with delight and also looked at me.

"He doesn't know how," the staff nurse suggested. "I'll do it for you."

"No, I want him to do it," she announced crossly, pointing at me.

"It's no problem," I boasted, taking her hand. "I have children of my own."

The nurses were doubtful and hovered over us, in the expectation I would need help.

Fortunately, the nappy was only wet.

Sarah was refusing to take a spoonful of medicine. I was called on to mediate.

"It's disgusting," she protested.

"But you do know that you need to take the medicine if you are to get better?"

"Well, why don't you taste some? It's horrible. You just try it."

"If I take it, will you?"

She nodded.

The syrup was absolutely foul.

I prescribed an alternative antibiotic which we both agreed was more palatable.

"Do you know Sheep Dip cures warts?"

"Sheep Dip?!"

"Yes, my dad put sheep dip on my warts and now they're gone."

I turned to his father, a farmer.

"Really? What is in sheep dip?" I had an idea it might contain organophosphate chemicals, which can have serious neurological side effects.

"No idea, but it's never done me any harm."

"It's definitely not a treatment I would recommend, but I'll check it out."

"Why is your nose purple like my Granda's?"

"I don't think my nose is purple."

Later, I found myself checking in a mirror.

Bigger questions

Jodie was almost 15 years old. She was a Jehovah's Witness, a Christian denomination. She would need a new kidney within months. We discussed all that was involved. As I expected, she wanted reassurance about one specific detail.

"Could I have the operation without getting any blood?" she asked.

For Jehovah's Witnesses, accepting a transfusion of donated blood - or even their own blood, collected and stored - goes against their beliefs. On the team, we considered how we might manage the surgery. I talked at length with Jodie's father to confirm his position regarding transfusion, and to receive his permission to discuss the matter in private with his daughter. First, I went over the situation with them together and, as expected, they were certain it was against God's law to receive another person's blood. Some weeks later, I had a chat with Jodie herself and concluded she had not been under undue pressure on the issue. She was an intelligent, thoughtful girl who recognised the risks of blood loss during major surgery. She talked with quiet confidence. Nothing from her cheery personality, trendy fashion choices, or artistic use of make-up, gave any indication of her personal religious beliefs.

The transplant surgeon was of the opinion that he should be able to perform the procedure with minimal blood loss. He could not, of course, give a cast iron guarantee. The anaesthetic staff weighed up the risks carefully. Once an operation is underway, the patient is fully their responsibility, including anaesthesia, pain relief, intravenous fluid management and blood transfusions. While respecting her beliefs they felt, on balance, that if a child's life was in danger, withholding a blood transfusion would cause them moral and professional difficulties.

A decision was made that the dilemma should be taken to the courts for guidance. In consideration of the paramount safety of the child, and her best interests, the court was asked to give authority for blood to be administered, should Jodie's life be at risk. Both sides, father, daughter, and the medical professionals, had their measured arguments presented.

I later learnt, from Jodie, that the judge invited her to visit his house and dine with his family, so that he might get to know her personally before declaring his ruling. In the relaxed atmosphere there, he asked her how she would feel if he was to find in favour of the anaesthetists. I was interested to learn of her response. She told me that she said to him, "I know you are a judge who must administer the law, and if that is what you decide, I know that is what you honestly feel you must do. I, however, do not believe I will need to be given blood, so you must do what you think is right, just as I am trying to do what is right for me."

I heard her repeat this story on several occasions, after she agreed to join a group of medical students in a discussion of such a dilemma as part of a medical ethics tutorial. The topic was patient autonomy. She always spoke confidently about the patient's right to make decisions about their own care. The students always left with a great respect for this young girl.

After careful consideration, the court ruled in favour of the anaesthetists. Despite this, Jodie gave her consent for the surgery to proceed.

On the day of her operation, I found myself calling into the operating theatre so frequently that the manager said kindly to me, "You know we will bleep you if any problem arises? You must have other patients to see?" I took the hint and left him alone.

I was present in the PICU when Jodie groggily regained consciousness. She looked frail against the white sheets. As she shifted into a more comfortable position, her eyes opened. Still woozy, she looked at the intravenous line in her arm. Then she looked at me and croaked: "Did I get any blood?"

"No, there was no need."

She managed a smile and whispered.

"I knew God would not let me have a transfusion."

Jodie reached out a hand to her dad as her eyes closed and she drifted off again.

Is the surgeon any good?

Jeremy was talking with the surgeon; the anaesthetist stood nearby with his parents. A nurse checked the name on his hospital wristband against her chart. I finished writing the clinical notes and handed them to the anaesthetist who reviewed the various blood test results with me and began to read through the file. When the surgeon finished talking with the boy, he turned to discuss the details of Jeremy's previous operations with his mother and father. Jeremy was looking anxious. He was old enough to understand that this operation was something he must go through but was worrying about how much pain he would have to endure and how long he would be in hospital. He was a strong lad but, just then, he felt ridiculous in the unattractive hospital gown and head gear.

When the transplant team left, I tried to calm his apprehension with a final chat. Fifteen minutes later, a scrub nurse appeared to escort him and his parents to the operating theatre. He delayed the move with a final question.

"Doc, is he a good surgeon?"

"Yes, he is the best transplant surgeon in Northern Ireland. You'll be in good hands."

I genuinely believed what I was saying. Satisfied with my response, off he went.

I always felt a certain anxiety and tension while the patient was out of my hands in the operating theatre but four hours later Jeremy was safely back in his bed. I checked his anti-rejection and analgesic drug prescription. The anaesthetist confirmed he was happy with his epidural which would keep Jeremy pain free until morning.

Some hours later, I was becoming concerned by a poor urine output and a deterioration in his renal function blood tests. I contacted the surgeon and he agreed an urgent scan was needed. I arranged it as I waited for him to join us. The scan suggested there was little blood flow through the graft.

"The kidney turned pink quickly once the clamps on the artery came off. There was definitely good perfusion of the kidney then."

The surgeon decided the boy must go back to theatre to have the kidney and the blood vessels supplying it examined directly. He was pessimistic.

When Jeremy heard this news, he was disgusted.

"You said he was the best!" he accused.

As he turned away from me towards his worried parent, I attempted to answer.

"That is why he is insisting on checking on his work."

This did not help.

A few hours later, I listened as our surgeon told me that the kidney had moved position internally after surgery was complete, even though he had considered this impossible as he closed up the wound. The change had resulted in a kink in one of the vessels, allowing a clot to form, which blocked the arterial supply. He had extracted the clot but the kidney had lost viability and it had been necessary to remove it. We were all enormously disappointed. It fell to me to speak to Jeremy.

He did not hold back.

"You promised me he was the best surgeon. Well, I think he is crap!" he shouted at me.

He refused to talk to the surgeon. Tears spilled from his eyes. I could only say how sorry I was, as I tried again to explain. Jeremy's parents, also dismayed, were embarrassed by his frank outbursts, but tried to buoy him up. They told him that the surgeon had promised he would go to the top of the waiting list for another kidney; that one would turn up, or they would give him one. He closed his eyes and sobbed. Soon, with a mixture of painkillers and exhaustion he succumbed to sleep.

Leaving the hospital a week later, and now back on dialysis, he still felt cheated. I felt the failure keenly. It would take some time to win back his trust.

Thankfully, we had the pleasure of seeing Jeremy in high spirits only a few months later, as headed home from a successful second transplant.

He made no comment on the surgeon this time.

When can I get out of here?

Roisin had been in hospital for a week. Her new kidney was proving slow to work at a satisfactory level. Several scans confirmed good blood flow through the organ. She herself was more concerned about how long she would be away from her home and her family. At first, she consoled herself that, at least for now, she did not need to attend secondary school. I sat on the side of her bed to explain something.

"For me to be sure the kidney will eventually work well, I need to perform a biopsy."

She looked at me from under her fringe of red hair, saying nothing, and awaited more details. She was at an age when communication with adults is kept to a minimum.

"It means going back to the operating theatre and having an anaesthetic. It is important you are perfectly still while I slip a needle into your new kidney so it's better if you are asleep for a few minutes and that way you will feel nothing. The biopsy needle takes a little core of tissue about the thickness of a pencil lead for analysis."

She looked at her aunt, who was with her that day to give her mother a chance to spend some time at home with her brother.

"If the doctor says it needs done, then it needs done".

Roisin shrugged, "Then will I be able to go home?"

I explained that we would examine the tissue in the laboratory and our findings would let us know what we needed to do to get the kidney working well enough for her to be discharged.

Resigned, she put her earphones back in and listened to Michael Jackson. Thriller was her favourite album.

"Whatever."

The biopsy showed no evidence of rejection, only temporary damage, known as acute tubular necrosis (ATN), resulting from the interruption to the kidney's blood supply while it was being transferred from the donor. This was relatively good news. Roisin's mum wanted to know how long recovery would take. Hearing it could be a week or more, Roisin was downcast again and withdrew into her music.

Just as all looked good at last, a urine infection caused a setback, resolved by a course of antibiotics and another week in hospital.

Despite clearing the infection, her blood tests indicated the kidney function had deteriorated again and another biopsy unfortunately suggested her body was starting to reject the transplant. Another delay. The anti-rejection drug regimen was adjusted with good effect.

Roisin rarely complained but sometimes I saw the sadness in her eyes. She was often wired for sound when I called to see her, but the nurses reported she perked up when she had new visitors, and that she enjoyed a bit of banter late at night.

On impulse, I called into a record store and bought a CD single I had heard on the radio. It was by a band called Chumbawamba and entitled Tubthumping. Next day, when we finished reviewing her, I produced it from my white coat pocket and handed it to Roisin. She read the label.

"Do you know the song?" I asked. She gave me a non-committal look and put it in her player.

"It made me think of you, putting up with being stuck here with us."

She put the buds in her ears again and pressed 'play'. I knew the opening words she'd be hearing as we moved on: "*I get knocked down, but I get up again, you are never gonna keep me down.*"

I gave a thumbs up, pointed at her and left. Later, as I passed by again, she waved, and her smile was back.

Afterwards at our ward meeting, sister, who was probably more up with pop music than me, asked, "You do know that song is about binge drinking?"

I was a little taken aback. The next time it came on the car radio I paid more attention to the rest of the hit and heard: "He takes a whiskey drink. He takes a vodka drink. He takes a cider drink. He takes a lager drink."

Uh-oh, I thought. Maybe not really appropriate for a 12-year-old.

The repetitive "I get up again" chorus cheered me up again, until a counter-melody gleefully boasted: "*Pissing the night away*".

I hoped the kidney would copy these latter words.

A few days later, I was relieved to see virtually normal results and Roisin surprised me.

"I have a present for you."

She removed a little box from her bedside drawer and handed it to me. It contained a slim silver pen. She took it back from me, rolled it over and held it up towards me. Inscribed on the side of the barrel were the words, "WHEN CAN I GO HOME?"

Two days later, her results were again fine. I said nothing but took the special pen from my top pocket. I opened her clinical file and noted the date then wrote in large capitals, "HOME TOMORROW."

I remarked, "this pen is a beautiful writer."

I turned the page around and showed it to her

She whooped and hugged her mum. The pen is still a treasured possession.

Does epo work on dogs?

Jonny ushered Sharon and their two children through the door. The busy Monday morning clinic was running late again. He showed no sign of irritation at having to wait past their appointment time, but instead greeted me with characteristic good humour,

"I bet you wish you had my faith healer here to help this morning."

We shared the joke, which dated back to when their little girl was born. Their son had been referred earlier when he was several months old because of cysts identified on a kidney scan at another hospital. We discovered that he had a rare genetic syndrome - but not before his sister was on the way. Fortunately, the boy's kidney function remained stable. After an antenatal scan, the new baby exhibited one of the signs of the same condition, multiple cysts in her kidneys. Although she passed urine soon after birth, her blood tests became progressively worse in succeeding days. The underlying syndrome was affecting her kidneys more severely than in her brother's case. It seemed she could not survive for many months without dialysis. I talked guardedly and as gently as possible with Jonny and Sharon about this option at such an early age. She was allowed home, affording them time to consider her future while we kept the infant under frequent review.

Unknown to me, her dad sought the help of a faith healer. This man, an ordinary farmer, was said to have "the gift." As the weeks went by, Caitlin's blood results gradually improved, which can actually happen in the rare condition with which the children were affected. We were delighted with her progress and eventually Jonny confided in me about visiting the healer. It was years before her kidney tests began to deteriorate again but, despite dietary restriction and supportive drugs, she would eventually need dialysis or a new kidney.

Her parents remained upbeat despite the demands of rearing two children with complex needs. Their mother continued to run her own business. Jonny was meticulous in the demanding care of the children and managed to continue his hobby of training racing greyhounds. I often met the loving grandparents who readily provided support when needed.

At the clinic, I usually got a detailed update of any new developments or difficulties since the previous visit. Admissions to the local hospital were not unusual. The parents were alert to behaviour changes which might seem minor to others, but which they recognised could be symptoms of a developing problem. Johnny often had pertinent questions as he assessed something that was worrying him. He was also an expert at using his sense of humour in an attempt to reduce the inevitable anxiety and tension which setbacks brought.

This morning, he had an unusual question for me.

"That EPO injection we give Caitlin to counteract anaemia," he began, "it's the same stuff professional cyclists have been caught using to help them go faster, isn't it?"

I confirmed this and pointed out that its supply was tightly controlled - which was why it was provided directly from the hospital pharmacy to Jonny. He appreciated that Caitlin needed it because her kidneys were no longer able to produce her own Erythropoietin, leading to anaemia. Epo, as he called it, raised her blood count, which gave her more energy and increased her general feeling of wellbeing.

Jonny effected to look around furtively.

"Does it work on dogs?"

I was aware of Hazel, the senior renal nurse, taking a deep breath behind me. Could he be serious? I set down my pen and looked at him. He leant forward.

"Somehow, we got a double delivery this month and I wouldn't like it to be wasted. I just was interested to know if it would work on the greyhounds."

As I sat considering a polite reply, Sharon interrupted.

"He's winding you up, doctor. You know what he's like."

He tried to keep a poker face, then roared with boisterous laughter, and slapped me on the shoulder. I could see that the sound was infectious as I looked at the children.

As I bid them goodbye later, the morning didn't seem quite so hectic.

Laughter, the best medicine

Ciaran was another father who enjoyed a joke, even at his own expense, but today he was not laughing. Like all fathers, he loved his daughter fiercely, undoubtedly more than anything else in his world, and she remained ill and in need of intensive care. When she was fearful, he specialised in distracting her by making her laugh with a funny story or a tickle. Perhaps this also acted as pressure release for his own anxiety. Rachel was diagnosed with a serious kidney problem early in infancy. She was now in PICU because the new kidney she received a few days before was not yet fully functional. As the ward round reached her bed, her mum and dad were at her side. The family became silent and watchful.

We reviewed her morning biochemistry results, and the overnight urine output with the intensive care staff. Rachel was quiet after the operation, in part because of the sedative effect of analgesia, but Ciaran was concerned that this was not the only reason she was not her usual happy, mischievous self.

We discussed our treatment options and I knew he was listening intently. To reassure him, I explained that transplanted kidneys do not always work immediately but gradually pick up over a few days, which was what was happening. He had probably been warned of this but may have forgotten.

"Rachel's blood results are improving steadily but her urine production is lower than I would like. A key part of our management is to balance her fluid intake with her urine output. We have to count up the volume of the intravenous drugs we are using, and then calculate how much she is allowed to drink. I appreciate how much restricting the amount we allow her to drink is upsetting her."

Ciaran confirmed this and patted his daughter's hand.

"She has been a great wee girl" added her mum. "She is so brave."

I decided to prescribe a drug called a diuretic. I reminded them that she had taken it before and that it should make her pass a lot more urine.

"What is it called doc?"

"It's called Lasix or Furosemide. Rachel's mum may remember giving it to her in the past."

"Is it an injection?" asked a little voice from the bed.

Her mum studied her hands, not sure of the answer. Ciaran's brow furrowed, then he smiled knowingly, as I reassured his daughter.

"No injection, Rachel, just a spoonful of medicine," I said.

He pointed at me, "Ah yes! That's the medicine you once secretly dropped in some of the nurses' tea for a laugh. It had them running to the toilet all day, so it should do the trick."

Having delivered this statement with a straight face, Ciaran watched the horror this untruth had caused to show on mine. The nurses, junior staff, and the senior intensivist looked at me with disbelief. I began an outraged denial.

Just then, Ciaran gave Rachel a gentle little nudge to let her know this was a grown-up joke, and broke into a laugh. I placed a hand on his shoulder and shook my head in resignation. His daughter rewarded him with a little smile.

"It was worth the lie, just to see your face," he grinned.

Rachel settled back into her pillows and closed her eyes, content to know her dad was in control.

Later in the tearoom, we discussed humour as a coping mechanism. I related how once, at a clinic, Ciaran advised me that if I wanted a good laugh, I should try secretly breaking a raw egg into someone's pint of Guinness.

"It's invisible there so they nearly always throw up when it slips into their mouth," he confided, clearly delighted at the memory.

Some months later, with his daughter now well, Ciaran informed me that with some friends, he was running the New York Marathon to raise money for the Children's Kidney Fund. Impressed, I asked how his training was going.

"Oh, not too badly. I play football regularly and train for that once or twice a week. I've also managed a few 10 kilometre runs."

As a seasoned marathon runner myself, I decided it was too late to suggest he should perhaps have built up his mileage to around 18 or 20 miles, to be sure he could manage the 26-mile course.

I met him again after the event when Rachel was extremely well and back at school.

"How did New York go?"

"It was a killer, but I did finish it. It took me six and a half hours. I could hardly walk the next day, I was so sore and stiff. Even climbing down the steps from the plane arriving back in Dublin was torture."

I made sympathetic noises.

"I gave Rachel the medal," he added.

Aaron's hug

Aaron was 10 or 12 years old when I first met him. He walked hesitantly into the room, taking shelter behind his mother and father. From behind this shield, he did not acknowledge me or respond to my greeting. Instead, he sat down in a corner and became absorbed in the screen of his electronic tablet. His parents explained that his behaviour was due to learning difficulties, which had been assessed and diagnosed when they lived in another part of the country. I heard that Aaron had no speech. He attended a special school where his needs were best met, and where he could receive the support he required. His mother coincidently worked in another part of the same school, which was a big help to his family. I concluded his disabilities would make communication between me and Aaron difficult. He had been diagnosed with a chronic kidney condition, unrelated to these other issues, and referred to the renal clinic. Clearly, his family was devoted to him.

Over succeeding months, I got to know him as a quiet, pleasant and at first uncommunicative boy. His kidney function was on a slow downward trajectory, which I discussed with his family. With Aaron, I tried to explain what I was doing as I examined him, and always warned him when I needed to take a blood sample. He appeared to take no interest in our conversations but acquiesced to various tests without protest.

Hospital visits took on a regular pattern and I dared to feel that I was gradually being accepted as part of his world.

On one occasion, I was surprised to learn from his father that not only was he quite skilled at the games his father had set up for him on the computer, but that he had managed to download a new one himself. I was to reflect on this some months later. Before that, his biochemistry readings gradually approached a critical level. The parents had been briefed on possible options and knew something of the other patients who attended the clinic. It was time to make difficult decisions, I informed them, "I'm afraid that without dialysis or a kidney transplant, we will not always have Aaron with us."

We looked at each other, and at Aaron, who was apparently engrossed in a game.

"We knew we would reach this point, sooner rather than later. We recognised where things were headed from his test results," said his father. They had thought ahead.

"We appreciate that there are more patients needing kidneys than the number of organs becoming available," his mother added. "We know Aaron would be competing with other children."

Without waiting for me to respond, they went on to mention one of my concerns.

"We just don't know how our lad would cope with the whole repetitive dialysis procedure. It could be enormously upsetting for him."

I was listening carefully and wondered what their conclusion might be.

"We would like to have our tissue types and Aaron's analysed. If you are agreeable, and providing one of us is a suitable tissue match, we would like to give him a kidney. What we want to know is, would it be possible to do the operation before he needs dialysis?"

I agreed to propose this to the transplant team. Pre-emptive live donor transplants were relatively unusual at the time.

There was further discussion of the pros and cons before all three family members had their blood drawn for testing. A few days later I delivered the results. It was good news. Next, I entered into discussions with the surgeon, the anaesthetists and the PICU staff. There was general acceptance and support for the plan.

I arranged for the family to meet the team, and for Aaron to visit the PICU. At the next clinic visit, we went through the usual routine, then I confirmed that both parents wished to proceed. They had no doubts. As they got ready to leave, I pointed out that we needed to think about how we would prepare Aaron, as we were unable to ask his opinion. Just then, he handed his tablet to his mum, stepped up to me, and briefly wrapped his arms around me.

"I think that was a 'yes'," said his dad

Aaron smiled and headed for the door. I realised that we were all smiling.

He was almost a perfect patient, both before and after surgery. He did not complain about intravenous drips or urinary catheters and the new kidney functioned early and well. Every one of us involved - nurses, doctors, and parents - were impressed and, admittedly, relieved.

I reflected that not only could Aaron download games for his tablet, but that he might be more sensitive than I appreciated. Indeed, he possibly understood more of what people said than he was able to easily express. I have not forgotten Aaron or what I learnt from knowing him - not least that children may be sensing a lot of what doctors and parents were discussing without understanding the details.

In 2022 while watching television coverage of the London Marathon I was surprised and delighted to see Aaron's parents run with a very happy boy in his racing wheelchair through the Elite start, and to learn later that they had completed the route.

Relief and release

Anyone whose child becomes ill, even with a simple viral infection, knows of the worry that can bring. A successful transplant therefore brings enormous relief to parents, often after years of anxiety. At last, they can see a future opening up for their child. The children are released from the constraints of repeated dialysis sessions to live a more normal life. For the nurses and doctors involved, there is a sense of fulfilment and a degree of elation each time. It is, of course, a team achievement.

I was once approached by a grandmother after a fundraising event.

"God bless your hands," she said, taking mine in her wrinkled ones.

I was deeply touched by these simple words. I tried to explain that I was not the surgeon but the medical nephrologist. This detail was unimportant to her. She was just grateful her grandson was well again. Her blessing was for all of us.

I sometimes asked the children, "What was the worst thing about having a kidney transplant?" The response could be surprising.

"When they flush the I/V after taking a blood sample. I hated that more than anything. That heparin stuff really stings, right up your arm."

Heparin is an anticoagulant solution, diluted in saline, used to prevent blood clotting in the line.

"What? Worse than the actual operation?"

"I was asleep for that," replied one girl.

"Well, you can thank our anaesthetist for that," I thought.

After I heard this grievance a number of times, I decided we needed to adjust the volume of Heparin, so that less could get in to irritate the vein.

Several mothers agreed that their worst moment was immediately before the surgery.

"I went into the operating theatre with my son, holding his hand as he lay on the table. I was encouraging him to be brave and trying to be brave myself. The anaesthetist was chatting and explaining to him what was happening and asked him to start to count down from 10. As he did so, the doctor attached a syringe to the I/V line and slowly advanced the plunger.

"Tom was holding my hand tightly. Ten, nine, eight, seven, six, he said quite clearly, then sleepily, five, four, three.

"I felt his hand go limp; his eyes rolled up. He was gone.

"I thought my own heart had stopped, I was paralysed but, with a nurse guiding me, I made it to the door. I could barely see it through my tears. I thought, 'Will he come through? Will he ever talk to me again?'"

I learnt a lot from such conversations. Mothers and fathers might be more frightened than their child but they often find the strength to suppress their feelings so they can concentrate on easing the little one's anxiety. The emotional cost is born of parental love and only offset by a successful treatment outcome.

Having an ill child can bring enormous stress for families. There is inevitable trepidation about the illness, treatment, and outcome. There may be financial pressures after having to take time away from work, on top of the disruption to family life, and the pressure on relationships with partners and other children. We were frequently impressed by how families battled through. Often help came as extended family and friends rallied in to support. Perhaps friendship and understanding from other families making, or who had made, the same journey is the best form of support. Nursing and medical staff often receive praise for the care they provide, but it is the mothers and fathers who deserve a medal.

It is almost 50 years now since I met Becky, who couldn't talk because of her tracheotomy. A few years later, I faced the plight of a child with advancing renal disease for whom there seemed no available treatment. Forty years ago, I supervised the first renal transplant of a young child in Belfast. We had started by dialysing small children with simple CAPD, running three or four bags of dialysis fluid in and out of the abdominal cavity each day. Now there are small, programmable peritoneal dialysis machines which are about the size of a carry-on flight suitcase. Indeed, they can be taken and used on holiday. The fluid required can be delivered to the holiday destination. While the modern machines perform continuous fluid changes overnight without interruption at the child's home, the efficiency or malfunction can be monitored remotely at the hospital. Haemodialysis has been available as an option for more than 30 years, even for the smallest child. For some, it can even be provided in the family home. The artificial kidneys employed have more biocompatible hollow fibre membranes, reducing the side effects of the process, and there is now a capacity to monitor biochemistry changes in real time. More often now, donated kidneys may come from living donors, usually from parents or relatives. The kidneys are removed by keyhole surgery allowing the donor to recover quickly. Some of our earliest patients have received a second and even a third kidney. This is possible thanks to advances in anti-rejection immunosuppressive drugs. It is therefore important to continue to pay great attention to the physical and mental health of patients.

Today's patients find it difficult to believe that, in the past, children and patients over the age of 55 were not accepted for renal replacement therapy. We have come a long way since then. Along the road, I have been moved by how ill children bring out the best in their parents and have learned a lot from both. I have been relieved and thrilled to see many patients return to an active, boisterous childhood.

Fit for anything

I watch as the eight amateur athletes line up in their lanes at the start line. They stand on the professional blue synthetic track, where some of their heroes have won national medals. The noise from their supporters in the Grandstand fades as the public address system crackles and announces the final of the 50 metre sprint for six to eight-year olds. The cheering crescendos, again and again, as each name is announced. It threatens to drown out the call for the runners to take their marks. The starter gun fires. The competitors leap forward and race down the track, some a little erratically.

These are the UK Transplant Games.

Each participant has had a lifesaving organ transplant. The Games have been held annually for 40 years across the UK, twice in Belfast. Hazel Gibson, our senior renal nurse specialist has organised (with some help) the team kit, the travel arrangements and accommodation, as efficiently as she organises the dialysis unit.

There are teams from every major paediatric centre in the country. Those from the major English cities may be large in number but our team, usually of around 10 children, can hold its own in terms of medals won, and supporter noise.

The children compete in five age bands, starting with the under-fives, rising up to the 15-to-17-year-old category.

The events cater for various levels of physical ability and include traditional track and field events, badminton, table tennis, football, and also tug of war, ball throwing, and an obstacle race.

For participants, competing on a level playing field brings a degree of sporting normality which, for some, may not be possible in a school setting. It is a pleasure to see the resulting boost in self-confidence and parental pride. Friendship and camaraderie develops between rivals, supporters and families, as they mix and share life experiences.

Above all, the games highlight the need for organ donation.

and Parents Deserve a Medal.

At the opening ceremony in Belfast, each team marches into the auditorium behind a standard. Each is met with enthusiastic cheering. One team generates the greatest response from the crowd, which rises in a prolonged standing ovation. But this team is not even competing. Their banner has two words emblazoned on it: "Donor Families". Some of the applause is mixed with tears.

Here, these people could see, for once, the tangible results of their generosity and humanity, at a time of personal tragedy and loss.

19. Funerals and weddings, endings and beginnings

I feel an enormous sadness, a great sense of loss and even a feeling of helplessness when I attend the funerals of children. The team will have tried everything we can but sometimes our best efforts are in vain. There is nothing more we can do now, except share in the family's grief. I pray they may find a way to cope. Family and friends, even parents of other patients, are often there to offer love and support. One morning, as I sit listening to a school choir singing softly in the background, I reflect on the joy this much-missed child will have brought in days gone by - first smiles, first words, first steps, first day at school. All around, folk sit or stand, faces unashamedly wet with tears. On occasion, I have been asked to read a passage from the Bible. This is a special privilege and I do so gladly, appreciative of the thoughtfulness behind the request. Some families find a measure of solace in their faith, which at such times provides them with an invaluable comfort. For others, the sense of loss may be just too great.

The drummer

At one farewell celebration, I was asked to say a few words about Christopher, a teenage boy who, after a long battle, had succumbed to a malignant lymphoma, a rare complication of immunosuppression. Every pew was full of people, old and young, pressed together, sitting in silence, or speaking only in whispers. Standing around the walls and at the rear of the room, every space was packed with his fellow pupils, all in school uniform.

Eventually, my time came to stand and speak of this special son, lost on the cusp of manhood. A boy who, like his father, loved to make music. I talked of a small boy with a shy smile that could brighten a room. From the lectern, I could see that some of his young friends were already in tears. My throat tightened in the charged atmosphere, and I was glad I written down what I planned to say. I paused after a few sentences to check my script and, as I looked up at the family, my voice weakened. I had a moment of panic that I might not be able to continue.

272

There came a crash as a schoolgirl fainted and slumped to the floor. In the brief pause while she was helped, I swallowed a mouthful of water and my voice recovered. The boy's schoolmaster and the father of another patient also spoke. When we all rise to file out, we are all deep in our own thoughts.

In the background, a song by the group REM , "Everybody Hurts", was playing, then I think,The Kinks -

Though you've gone, you're with me every single day, believe me.

Sisters

Patients in the PICU are inevitably critically ill. Thankfully, for most, if not all, of their stay they are likely to be unaware. Not so the anguished parents, watching their sedated and ventilated child; nor the staff, knowing that their every decision or action may be crucial to the child's survival. Supporting families is as much part of intensive care as the high-tech equipment and the medical management of life-threatening conditions. Many nurses eventually elect to move on to less demanding positions, as the pressure of the work and the recurrent loss of patients takes its toll. For others, the motivation to continue comes from the pleasure of seeing a child discharged from the unit, rescued from the very brink of death.

On occasions, you have the privilege of experiencing unique moments that are both humbling and uplifting.

After battling to save a child for many weeks, I reached a point of knowing we had lost the fight. Sarah was a girl who was born with numerous problems, making her future seem precarious when she was tiny - but by now she had a history of defying doctors, and even proving them wrong. Her family - mother, father and two other girls - were very close. They had cared for her and fought for her all her life. As a result, against the odds, she attended school, loved her life, and developed an independent spirit and mind of her own, despite her many disabilities. I had got to know her and respect her family and, because of her limited understanding, continued to monitor her kidney problems past the usual age limits of the children's hospital. Eventually, the time came when we agreed she should transfer to an adult clinic near their home and, regretfully, I said goodbye.

273

Some time later, her family contacted me again. Sarah's kidneys had continued to deteriorate. They were distressed that, because of her complex needs and disabilities, they were convinced that she was not being considered for renal replacement therapy. They asked that she might come back under my care. I could understand this request but was faced with a dilemma regarding her age and that she was another doctor's patient. I appreciated that her parents wanted their girl to be treated as an individual in her own right. I needed to weigh up all sides of the situation carefully, not just one aspect.

"You know her so well," her parents protested. "Each of us loves her and she gives back three times the love in return. It is so hurtful to hear that she is not worthy of a kidney transplant."

I agreed to bend the rules to see her again, although I was reluctant to give any guarantees for the future. Her care passed back to me.

Surprisingly, a suitable kidney did become available for which there was no competition from another patient. Her parents had no hesitation in handing her over to the transplant team. In the succeeding days and weeks, several postoperative complications developed. Despite further surgery, and intensive treatment, her situation became precarious.Now I was sitting with her family trying gently to tell them what they already knew. We had run out of options. They had no regrets and were grateful that their daughter had been given every chance. A short time later, their mother and father informed me that her sisters had a special request.

"When Sarah was ill at home, we would get into bed beside her to comfort her. We loved to do that for her." I looked at them, picturing the scene. Their eyes appealed to me and to Sarah's nurse, "Do you think we could get in beside her one last time?"

The airway tubing, intravenous lines and the wiring of the electronic monitors were carefully moved aside. Sarah was wrapped in her sisters' arms. We moved screens around the bed and left them all together.

Going home

My footsteps echoed through the cavernous multi-storey car park. It was virtually empty at this late hour of the evening. Leaving the cold and silent building, I walked through the darkness of the winter night. Soon, I passed the vacant reception area, crossed the empty entrance hall and headed for the elevator. The machinery groaned as it slowed. "Third-floor, oncology and haematology," announced a lifeless, robotic voice. With a heavy heart, I stopped outside a side room door. I was thinking about the phone call I had received a few hours earlier, telling me that one of my old patients was terminally ill. The message diverted me from returning to the warmth and comfort of home. I suspected I would not be reading bedtime stories to my daughters that night. Entering quietly, I stood for a moment as my eyes adjusted to the gloom. I registered the green glow of the cardiac monitor. My own heart pounded, my eyes stung, I felt the skin on my neck and arms prickle.

Róisin was lying still on the bed, her eyes closed, held in comfort by crisp, white sheets. In the dim light of the angle-poise lamp, her skin was white, her lips pale, her breathing almost imperceptible, but she seemed strangely peaceful as she slept. I became aware that her mother and father had risen to their feet behind me. I turned towards them and involuntarily stretched out my hands. Her mother stepped into my arms. We held onto each other in shared grief. I raised my eyes and looked over at the big man standing there, for once, looking helpless. I held out my right hand to him, and it was taken in a strong rough grip and turned into a bear-like hug. Tears spilt down his unshaven face.

"Thank you for coming," he whispered.

My throat was so painful that, at first, I was unable to speak. I shook my head, searching for words. I knew that the girl's stepfather loved her as much as any father, loved her as his own. As if reading my thoughts, he spoke, filling the silence.

"You know how fond she was of you."

Again, I struggled to reply ,"She was always a very special little girl to me," I managed to say at last. "She didn't say a lot to me when she was small, and I was still a stranger to her. Growing up she rarely complained, not about blood tests, not about operations, I think she only cried when she wanted to go home. We got to know each other so well. When she got older though, I had to scold her a few times, because I suspected she wasn't taking her tablets regularly. She could turn on a good sulk," I smiled ruefully, "I hope she understood it was because we cared about her so much."

Her mother answered softly in the darkened room

"She never held it against you when you seemed cross. She might never have admitted it, but in her own way she looked forward to coming up to the clinic in Belfast, especially when she was so well, after getting her new kidney."

We stood together looking at Róisin, now a young woman, each with our memories. I thought of the baby girl with the red-brown hair, her dark eyes that spoke even before she could form many words; of the night, I found mother and daughter - or was it aunt and niece? - asleep, side by side, arms around each other, both in the metal hospital cot; of the schoolgirl, smart in her new uniform; of her love of pop music; and of the brave teenager faced with weeks of chemotherapy. I felt anger and despair at how unfair life could be.

I tried to lighten the moment, "She wasn't too pleased when I vetoed her having her ears pierced because of the risk of infection with the drugs she was taking."

"Nor when you said an eyebrow ring wasn't a great idea either," replied her mother with a little smile. "Then she came up with the idea of a nose stud. She was just being a normal 14-year-old, enjoying life, and enjoying winding us up. She beat us all in the end. More power to her. That was one of our last visits to the children's clinic. She was so full of life. I will never forget the look on your face when she pulled up her sleeve to show you that tattoo of Michael Jackson on her shoulder!"

A little voice came from the bed.

"You said I had got too big for the outpatient Wendy House." The old cheeky smile flickered on her face. I walked over and sat down on her bed wondering how long she'd been listening. Her mum lifted her up a little and held her.

"I knew you would come."

Gently, I took her right hand in mine and gave it a little squeeze.

"Was I one of your favourite patients then?" she whispered.

"Doctors aren't allowed favourites," I answered with a smile.

Our eyes met and I leant over to brush a kiss on her forehead, then whispered in her ear, "Yes, of course you were."

Her mum and dad sat down on the other side of her bed and shortly her hand slipped from mine. Just then, an attentive ward auxiliary nurse quietly looked in. "I've got some tea and biscuits next door."

We sipped the tasteless hospital brew, reminiscing over the good days and tough days we had shared when Róisin was a child; and about all she had been through in recent months.

Eventually I said, "No matter what happens, she has known nothing but love from both of you and her brother and her favourite aunt Marie." I paused, "Let's go back in and see her again, then I should leave you with her and head home."

As we rose, Róisin's mother, June, turned to me, "She's not going to make it this time, is she?"

The choking ache was back in my throat.

"No, I don't think so," I agreed sadly.

"I think she knows that," said her dad, "and she knew you would come."

The death of a child is the worst catastrophe that can happen in anyone's life. Parents are devastated, hurting and heartbroken; brothers and sisters grief-stricken, distressed and confused as they try to understand what has happened. Parents have come to the doctors saying, "our little girl or little boy is seriously ill, can you please help?" And we do everything we possibly can but, sadly, we do not always succeed.

I have emphasised that paediatric medicine is a partnership between doctors, nurses and others, working together with parents to do the very best we can for sick children. Over time, these children become, at an emotional level, part of an extended family for each of us on the hospital team. Emotions can, of course, influence decisions - but as professionals we endeavour to act not just compassionately, but rationally. We avoid the temptation of offering comforting, but overly optimistic outcome predictions. Those may only lead to unrealistic expectations, and possibly bitter disappointment.

The death of any of our patients upsets every member of the team. For me, there is an acute and indescribable sense of loss, but for the family, the pain never goes away. Parents have told me that when you lose a child, a part of you goes with them. Someone has said that when old people die, we bury them in the ground but when we lose a child, we bury them in our hearts.

A wedding present

The father of the bride rose to his feet and removed some notes from a pocket. Loud applause bounced off the ceiling and around the ballroom. The good-natured cheering and whistling gradually died down and the room quietened. The big man looked down at the lovely young woman beside him. He tried to speak but was overcome by emotion.

Some 20 years ago, when she was only approaching four years of age, he gave his little girl a kidney. Today at the church, in the old tradition, he had given her away to her childhood sweetheart

This was the biggest wedding Anne and I ever attended. We had driven to Hilltown, along a winding road at the foot of the Mourne Mountains. The car park was already almost full, as was the church, when we arrived. Soon there was not an empty pew. After the ceremony, Megan delighted the throng outside as she bounced from guest to guest. Her beautiful dress was only outshone by the happiness on her smiling face.

"What about you, Dr Savage? How's it going, Anne?" she laughed, as we exchanged hugs.

Now, at the hotel reception, her father struggled to say a few words. Megan reached a hand towards him and her brother gently took his notes. Between the two men, the speech was delivered. Everyone rose to toast the bride and groom. Then it was the groom and best man's turn, each greeted with heckles and a standing ovation, and followed by the appropriate toasts. Just as everyone thought it was time for the food, and perhaps more drink before the dancing, the bride's mother stood up. Paula signalled for silence.

"There are some people here today who we are especially pleased to have with us. People without whom Megan might not be here."

278

At our table is Colette, a nurse who looked after Megan not just in hospital, but as a willing babysitter, even when she was on home dialysis. We began to get embarrassed and apprehensive as she continued.

"At Megan's clinic visits, her doctor always wrote in her hospital notes with a silver fountain pen. As a toddler, Megan set her heart on getting her hands on that pen, so that she could try it out. It made no difference if she was warned not to touch it. When Megan sets her mind on something, she usually succeeds, as her husband will find out. Dr Savage developed a strategy to save his pen from destruction. He kept a supply of plastic ball point pens in his desk, which he would try to give to her instead."

I grinned at the forgotten memory of those battles. She never wanted the cheap substitutes, sometimes even crossly throwing them on the floor.

"As a thank you for his care over the years, we want to give him something tonight. Something which Megan has picked specially."

She then presented me with a beautiful fountain pen which I treasure and have been using as I write this story.

There is one thing, however, which gave me more pleasure than the pen; the birth of Megan and Dermott's baby boy, Tadhg, a year or two later.

The mitt of St Jude

Once Ronan had led Ciara unto the floor, the music and dancing had taken over the evening. I sat watching the impromptu but expert choreography triggered by an upbeat Country and Western number. It was clearly a favourite of the wedding guests but completely unknown to me. Lines of lads and girls, women and men, swayed back and forward, performing in unison, complex movements of their hands, legs, feet and bodies. Enormously impressed, I recognised that the level of coordination required would be well beyond my capabilities. The song ended to wild applause and a cheer. A few of the game, older and more overweight performers collapsed back, sweating into their chairs, to summon replacement fluids. Already, another favourite had the floor full again. I found myself pulled to my feet by good-natured dancers and lost myself in the rhythm and happiness of the night. I was reminded of an old Irish saying, "There are no strangers here, only friends you've yet to meet."

Earlier in the day, at the long, traditional wedding mass, I was grateful, as an outsider, for the detailed printed guide to the ceremony. The key men arrived dressed in expensive matching suits, apparently relaxed, and having a bit of craic as the clock ticked slowly past the appointed hour.

At last, the glowing bride entered in a spectacular white dress, undoubtedly nervous, but showing no visible signs of this, thanks to the support of her bridesmaids, who charmed everyone, laughing over the length of that customary delay. Seeing her approach on her father's arm, the groom involuntarily developed an enormous smile.

The priest now brought an appropriate air of solemnity to the proceedings with a somewhat ponderous delivery. As we moved through the liturgy, I became aware that a group of rather irreverent lads in the pew behind us were following the Saturday afternoon football scores in the Premier League on their smartphones, more closely than the main event in the Chapel. At last, after virtually everyone, including the football supporters, had gone forward to participate in the Eucharist, the priest relaxed and invited the new husband to kiss the bride. This was greeted with delighted applause, whoops and cheers from the entire congregation. Following the throng, we exited into the autumn sunshine to shower the couple with rice and confetti.

It was wonderful to have been invited to share the day and now, late into the evening, the groom's father, a good friend, joined our table. We reminisced about the days we first got to know each other, when his son had been a seriously ill toddler. Now, as he was about to become a married man, he had decreed that his past illnesses and kidney transplants were not to be mentioned in any of the speeches. Today was to be about him and Ciara and their future together, not the past.

This was always a family who played down the demands and sacrifices his treatment entailed. I, of course, was aware of the difficult, worrying and sometimes frightening days they had faced with faith and courage. The kidney that had carried him healthily through to his wedding day was found through the generosity of his father - who had donated one of his own kidneys in a three-way swap, co-ordinated across the country. It was rapidly transported and transplanted into a patient in another unit, with whom he was an excellent tissue match. Simultaneously, the relative of another

280

patient also donated a kidney and as a result, within hours, Ronan was able to receive an equally well-matched organ.

As the celebrations waxed and waned around us, I confessed that the problems we had faced with Ronan's first transplant had taught me crucial lessons which benefited many succeeding patients. In the months after the surgery, he had been plagued by recurrent urinary infections. Particularly nasty bacteria proved difficult to eradicate. Eventually, we came to understand that the underlying problem was poor bladder function, which was only resolved by further surgery. Infection is potentially life-threatening in children whose immune system is suppressed by the drugs that counteract the body's normal inclination to reject foreign organs. Achieving a balance between eradicating an infection and threatening the viability of a new kidney is a major challenge for the medical team. Subsequently, I was more meticulous in identifying such bladder dysfunction pre-operatively, a task which became easier as more sophisticated urodynamic imaging techniques were developed.

Our talk moved on to the events of the day. The family and the groom, it was clear, were delighted and moved by the religious ceremony and in particular by the ministration of the presiding priest. I learnt he was not, in fact, the local Parish Priest, but a person who had a special connection with the family. Indeed, I heard that, despite being ill himself, he had been determined to take up their invitation to officiate.

"You may not remember this, but the second kidney Ronan received almost 17 years ago initially refused to work. Even after the second day, while you kept reassuring us that transplanted kidneys take time to function. You explained this is usually a consequence of being deprived of a blood supply and frozen when packed in ice during transport from one hospital to another."

"Yes, I know those are anxious hours - and not just for patients and families but for us in the team," I agreed.

Ronan's father continued, "I have a confession to make. We were not completely convinced that all would work out well, despite your reassuring words. We didn't want to question your expertise too openly, but, increasingly worried, we decided to get some input from a higher authority".

I looked at him with surprise. This was all news to me.

"We could see for ourselves that the volume of urine being passed and recorded was no greater than it had been before the operation, despite your optimism and our prayers. We talked to our local priest, who had been a source of strength to us on many occasions in the past, and he promised to visit the hospital. He arrived late in the evening to see our boy and brought with him a precious holy relic - The Mitt of St. Jude. Now I know what happened next may be something beyond medical science, and difficult to accept rationally."

The groom's father kindly laid a hand on my arm. He now had my full attention and that of others at the table.

The music, although still blasting, was no longer a distraction.

"Well, he laid the mitt on Ronan and prayed with us for divine intervention, and shortly afterwards he left."

He paused.

"By morning, urine was flowing freely down the catheter and into the measuring burette and drainage bag. Indeed, eventually so much was being passed, that you prescribed extra intravenous fluids to keep pace with the output."

As he said this, his thoughtful face broke into a smile.

"I'm not sure which of us was happier. But I'm telling you all of this now, because that was the same priest who blessed the bride and groom today."

A few years later I was delighted to hear that Ronan and Ciara had a beautiful baby daughter, Hollie, and more recently a son, Matthew.

Good memories

It is a widely accepted belief that the traumas of early childhood affect our entire adult lives. I like to think that good memories from those early days may equally offer protection in times of adversity. My reason for hoping this comes in part, from conversations I have had with patients who have grown into adulthood.

"What do you remember of your transplant operation all those years ago?" I have asked with some trepidation, not sure what the response might be. One young man, whom I now count as a friend, answered by opening a few buttons on his shirt.

"If I didn't have this big scar, I would almost believe it never happened."

It was his answer that led me to ask others. Of course, I knew he was still attending an adult clinic for follow-up blood tests - and I knew from experience that his parents could describe the events around his surgery in minute detail. He had listened to them relate the story many times and believed every word they said.

Those were days they would never forget.

I accept that it is possible that people forget scary or painful experiences by involuntarily confining them to some inaccessible part of their consciousness - a sometimes useful self-protection that makes old traumatic events bearable.

Probing further, it became clear that my former patient remembered more than he initially let on.

"What about all those blood tests you had back then?"

He screwed up his face.

"I detested needles of course, but doesn't everyone?"

I had to agree. He looked thoughtful, then amused.

"I do know my mother was always there," he grinned. "I even remember her talking about being able to see the male doctor's underpants. She noticed they could just be seen through a gap where the trousers of the surgical scrubs were tied together, like pyjamas, except at the side, over the hip. Her comments weren't always complimentary. She claimed one older doctor's pants were so washed out that they were grey rather than white. Some fancier ones, she classified as sexy. She was such an embarrassment. I was horrified that one of them might hear."

I admitted that I actually knew about this game at the time, and we laughed about it. I recognised her love was expressed in a little bit of rude humour, designed to distract a small boy. In doing so, she had created a good memory under stressful circumstances.

I have discovered recently that Fyodor Dostoyevsky agrees with me when he says, in *The Brothers Karamazov*, "There is nothing higher, stronger and more wholesome, and good for life in the future, than some good memory of childhood. If one carries such memories into life, one is safe to the end of one's days, and if one has only one good memory left in one's heart, even that may be the means of saving us."

While it seems unlikely that many of us on the renal team have ever read these words, I know that each one - nurse specialists, social workers, play therapists, psychologists, ancillary staff, parents, and doctors - go out of their way daily to give the children in our care good memories to mitigate the painful and unpleasant aspects of the treatment they experience. Children need to feel safe and comforted, especially when unwell. Hospitals are not cozy places, so cuddles from mum, dad and people they trust are important.

Science is the basis for the practice of modern medicine and nephrology, and its application underpins our foremost aim, to return our patients to health. But kindness and gentleness are at the heart of paediatric practice, complemented by compassion, a sense of humour and a friendly listening ear.

Being with families at times of crisis has an emotional cost, as the balance between self-belief and self-doubt is tested, but I never found myself asking, "Why am I doing this job?" Rather, I consider it a privilege to have had the opportunity to contribute to saving, and improving children's lives.

Acknowledgements

I wish to thank friends and colleagues without whom the renal replacement programme for children could not have been developed. The medical staff and nurses from the adult unit at Belfast City Hospital who took the children into their hearts in those early days: Joyce Weyl, Brid Thompson, Joanne Brown and Suzanne Scott among them. The transplant and paediatric surgeons who worked together: Robert Kernohan, John Connolly, Victor Boston and Stephen Brown.

Thanks to all our very special paediatric renal nurses: Joyce Gardener (sadly no longer with us), Joanne Sharrat, Hazel Gibson, Rosi Simpson and others. Thanks too, to my highly valued and supportive friend and consultant paediatric nephrology colleague of many years, Mary O'Connor.

Thanks to readers of early versions of book. Some chapters were offered to the creative writing and memoir group at the Crescent Arts Centre in Belfast. Their comments, advice and criticism and that of our mentor, Jo Egan, were invaluable. Thanks to my friends Joe Miles and Peter Robinson, and to family members Joanna, my daughter, and Jane, my niece, who were first readers of the completed manuscript. I would also like to acknowledge Seán O'Halloran of Clachan Publishing for his editorial advice and to thank him for getting this book to print.

A very special thanks to my son, Mark, who read and critiqued several drafts, and provided expert grammatical and structural advice. He has skilfully edited the final version.

Most of all, thank you to all the young patients and parents I have met over some forty years. Many have generously given permission for their stories to be told. While all the stories are true, or at least based on fact, with the passage of time, I have not been able to contact others. Where this is the case, I have changed names, locations and details in an effort to preserve confidentiality.

I hope their tales will inspire some young people to study medicine, perhaps even aspire to be paediatricians and to practice Medicine for service more than reward.